# GERIATRIC PSYCHOLOGY

## A BEHAVIORAL PERSPECTIVE

# GERIATRIC PSYCHOLOGY

## A BEHAVIORAL PERSPECTIVE

Richard A. Hussian, Ph.D.

Department of Psychology
University of North Carolina at Greensboro

 **VAN NOSTRAND REINHOLD COMPANY**

NEW YORK   CINCINNATI   ATLANTA   DALLAS   SAN FRANCISCO
LONDON   TORONTO   MELBOURNE

Van Nostrand Reinhold Company Regional Offices:
New York  Cincinnati  Atlanta  Dallas  San Francisco

Van Nostrand Reinhold Company International Offices:
London  Toronto  Melbourne

Library of Congress Catalog Card Number: 80-29701
ISBN: 0-442-21916-4

Manufactured in the United States of America

Published by Van Nostrand Reinhold Company
135 West 50th Street, New York, N.Y. 10020

Published simultaneously in Canada by Van Nostrand Reinhold Ltd.

15  14  13  12  11  10  9  8  7  6  5  4  3  2


Library of Congress Cataloging in Publication Data

Hussian, Richard A.
  Geriatric psychology.

  Bibliography: p.
  Includes index.
    1. Geriatric psychiatry. 2. Aged—Psychology.
3. Behavior therapy. I. Title. [DNLM: 1. Be-
havior—In old age. 2. Behavior therapy—In old
age. 3. Models, Psychological. 4. Psychology—
In old age. WT 150 H972g]
RC451.4.A5H87      618.97'689      80-29701
ISBN 0-442-21916-4      AACR1

*To my wife, Melanie,*
*and my brother, Bill.*

# Preface

This book was instigated, covertly rehearsed, and finally written due to a concern involving three existing deficiencies. The first deficiency was the observation that individuals who make up the sizable geriatric population were not adequately considered in the literature or the practice of psychology. In my own clinical work with elderly clients a rather pervasive anxiety was present throughout the assessment and treatment process. This anxiety appeared to be associated with what may best be described as a lack of certainty which, in turn, was derived from the recognition that significant differences existed between this population and the populations more widely described throughout my training and in the literature. The populations most studied, those of children and neurotic adults, offered useful frameworks, but provided little in the specificity needed. It became increasingly obvious that there were considerations which were unique to the geriatric situation that necessitated special attention.

Second, much of what was documented as representative of elderly behavior was written by thoughtful academic psychologists. Their scholarly input, though much needed in the early stages of a newly developing field, was somehow several levels removed from the problems most often confronted in the applied setting. Something can be said for a collection of observations from a clinical perspective, whether presented in a scholarly fashion or not. Although it was recognized that the flow of information in any field which enjoys both theoretical and applied components usually is unidirectional, I saw no reason for a continuation of this bias in an area which was young enough to avoid the errors of more established fields. The dual contingencies which control the behavior of professionals in these two camps (academic versus applied) could only result in a model in which the essential ingredient of feedback was missing.

Third, those few observations which were documented by predominately clinically oriented professionals also tended to be less than satisfactory. In this case, though, it was not the direction which was unsatisfactory, but rather that these observations were obtained by less than rigorous methods. Here was an ideal opportunity to establish reliable relationships quite early and to avoid inferential leaps, and yet these early clinical reports were generally couched in psychodynamic or otherwise loose terminology. This was certainly not in keeping with a science of behavior. It was also apparent that my behavioral colleagues were, perhaps, finding the waters rough going while attempting to remain attached to their theoretical supports.

It follows then that someone who has the unmitigated egotism to think that he or she can bridge the gaps between scientific constructs and application, and between organic concerns and behavioral responses, should undertake such an enterprise. It appears that by viewing typically documented responses of the elderly in terms of compensatory behavior rather than as irreversible ravages of aging may be an effective mechanism for explaining geriatric behavior. It remains to be seen whether or not this enterprise was, indeed, successful. If not, it is hoped that the *presentation* will be blamed and not the concept. It seems that man can have his format criticized and still function but to have his whole perspective scoffed at tugs at his credibility too much.

Many persons contributed indirectly to this book by shaping conceptual thinking and by disciplining presentation skills. Drs. P. Scott Lawrence and Cheryl Logan were most instrumental in this regard.

More directly, I wish to thank Elizabeth Hunt for her splendid work on the manuscript; Dr. H. R. Parker, Marie Miller, F.N.P., and Gale Harkness, P.A., for sharing their medical knowledge; Larry Long, R. Ph., Richard Ward, R. Ph., and Wanda L. Lovette, R. Ph., for sharing their pharmacological knowledge; James R. Saylor and the entire staff of The Evergreens for having patience with me during the writing of this book; and Melanie Spence for providing encouragement and the perfect atmosphere.

To the patients of The Evergreens go my deepest appreciation, for without them I would not have even noticed that a deficiency existed.

Richard A. Hussian, Ph.D.,
Department of Psychology,
University of North Carolina at Greensboro.

# Contents

# 1
# The Nature
# of the Population

Any decisions regarding the therapeutic process with a particular age group depend upon reliably collected data concerning that group's "normal" functioning. Clinical intervention in childhood disorders, for example, is at least partially based upon the knowledge of natural development in the early years. Decisions regarding whether or not to intervene, what behaviors are statistically normal for one age range but not another, and what level of functioning is the desired post-treatment criterion are related to empirically obtained data with children as subjects.

This relation between experimental findings and clinical application is not as well documented with the elderly. This deficit may be due to the crystallization thought to occur in senescence and the resultant lack of modifiability. The majority of early experimental findings have been based upon institutionalized samples of the elderly and these pessimistic results have made most clinicians, until very recently, hesitant to intervene in the problems of the aged. To view aging as progressive and irreversible deterioration due to naturally occurring organic processes would inevitably lead to programs of custodial care only. To recognize that certain changes do consistently occur, however, provides a standardized norm from which to work. It is necessary, then, to view problematic behavior of the elderly patient against the backdrop of correlated, normal changes.

This chapter presents empirically gathered data with the elderly as subjects in order to summarize the deficits which are present, to lend support to a new model of aging, and to set the stage for the accurate assessment and treatment of geriatric disorders. The usual inclusion of a section describing, statistically, the intense need for clinical intervention with this population will be omitted since such an argument would be redundant at this time and, hopefully, unnecessary.

## EXPERIMENTAL FINDINGS WITH THE ELDERLY

There are several dangers in the interpretation of empirical studies which use elderly subjects. First, it is difficult to sample randomly from the population of elderly persons since they are relatively more wary of participation in experimental research than other age groups. The elderly persons who were captive subjects, however, upon which a majority of the early research was conducted, were residents in nursing homes, homes for the aged, and mental hospitals. The results from these early studies are partially responsible for the hesitancy involved in the psychological treatment of the aged individual. Second, differential performance on a variety of experimental tasks is used in these studies to show age-related deficits. Two or more groups with disparate mean ages are compared on any number of dependent measures with statistically significant differences a frequent result. It should be noted that such cross-sectional experimentation does not verify deterioration in performance with advanced years. Aging is not the only pre-experimental difference between groups. Educational, cultural, and linguistic differences, among others, are potential confounds. Third, the interaction of psychological and physical difficulties in this age range is most acute. The incidence of cardiovascular disease, chronic heart failure, arteriosclerosis, atherosclerosis, hypertension, chronic renal failure, sensory impairment, cancer, and consumption of medication for these and other problems is much higher among the elderly than any other age group. These physical conditions, with their concomitant psychological aspects, are difficult to equate between groups. Bias is present even when dealing with noninstitutionalized elderly samples since the members of this cohort tend to have more physical handicaps, rely more on financial support from others, have higher unemployment rates, depend more on other family members for activities of daily living, are more often widows and widowers, and have attended fewer years of school than other age groups. These differences inherent in sampling are also, in part, responsible for the complication of clinical processes. Despite these limitations, however, some general trends are fairly reliable and may serve the basis of providing normative data for the geriatric clinician.

## SENSATION AND PERCEPTION

The elderly person is often stereotyped as a slow-moving, fragile skeleton, whose senses have dulled and whose perceptions are distorted. The overall slowing of response times commonly reported in almost all performance tasks have often been explained in terms of a deterioration of sensory mechanisms or in the process of perception. If these sensory systems should prove to be atrophied to a great degree, it should be reasonable to expect a general slowing in response time as well as the often documented increase in depressive reactions due to altered and/or reduced input. Indeed, the research in the areas of sensation and perception indicate reductions in sensitivity to external stimuli, but these decreases appear to be minimal. Decreased sensitivity has been reported with vibratory thresholds (Kenshalo, 1977), speech and speech discrimination (Corso, 1977), in the perception of verticality (Lawton & Nahemow, 1973), visual acuity (Anderson & Palmore, 1974), visual and auditory thresholds, light accommodation, blue-green differentiation, and dichotic digit span (Birren et al., 1963). There is also an increase in the incidence of presbycusis (high tone loss) and presbyopia (farsightedness), as well as a poorer level of dark adaptation, a decrease in the critical fusion threshold, a decline in contrast sensitivity, an increase in the Weber ratio in both the visual and auditory modalities (Fozard, Wolf, Bell, McFarland, & Podolsky, 1977; Spencer & Dorr, 1975), a decrease in stereopsis (Jani, 1966), and a deficit in the utilization of binaural direction cues (Warren, Wagener, & Herman, 1978). Elderly subjects also have more difficulty ignoring irrelevant information in visual search tasks (Rabbitt, 1968). However, no changes have been found in temporal discrimination thresholds in hearing, the speech feedback mechanism (Birren et al., 1963), olfactory sensitivity (Rover, Cohen, & Shlapack, 1975), or vigilance behavior (Davies & Griew, 1965). Decreases in susceptibility to many optical illusions are also reported (Lawton & Nahemow, 1973).

The reductions in sensitivity and sensory processing mentioned above are very slight, especially among the nonphysically ill elderly. Interpretation of these small age differences must be tempered by considering the experimental setting and the demand characteristics of the laboratory arrangement. These slight age differences are attributable, in part, to factors other than those brought about by aging. Whenever time is taken to increase the elderly subjects' familiarity with the equipment or the task requirements such as through practice, the age decrement is reduced even more (e.g., Hertzog, Williams, & Walsh, 1976). Also, when the motivation to respond accurately is increased the elderly tend to perform more like younger subjects.

In summary, there are slight age differences in some measures of sensory sensitivity and perception as shown in cross-sectional studies, but these differences are minor and do not lend support to the notion that response speed slowness is due to dysfunctions of peripheral mechanisms. Given the proper motivation, familiarity, and time to make a response, older healthy individuals perceive information almost as well as younger individuals. Therefore, the differences in overt behavior (output) often observed in the elderly are not primarily due to single-mode losses of information at the receptor or processing levels. However, the multiplicity of these slight deficits across modalities may result in a behavioral picture of significant overall decline.

## LEARNING AND MEMORY

Until recently, the adage regarding old dogs and learning was considered a truism. To work under this assumption, however, would severely limit any learning-based treatment strategy in favor of a maintenance or medication approach. It would also be impractical to teach skills or condition responses in therapy only to have this knowledge forgotten. Studies in the area of learning and memory suggest that such assumptions are not entirely warranted.

Shmavonian, Miller, and Cohen (1968) have shown that classical conditioning with elderly persons is more difficult than with younger persons, but that these age differences become insignificant when the intensity of the unconditioned stimulus is increased. On the other hand, Botwinick (1967) found that the conditioned response extinguished more rapidly in older subjects than younger ones. This more rapid extinction rate appears to be correlated with difficulty in acquisition of the conditioned response. It has also been shown that older subjects' galvanic skin responses show quicker habituation to a conditioned stimulus alone (Botwinick & Kornetsky, 1960). These results suggest that, in clinical behavioral applications, conditioned emotional responses such as in avoidance or escape, learning may take longer to develop and, once established, may necessitate more continual pairings (in the form of booster sessions) even after intervention has terminated.

As minor as the age differences found in classical conditioning are, there are even less significant age differences with an operant conditioning paradigm. However, acquisition is still considered to take longer and there is also an age difference in the resistance to extinction. This time, however, the older subjects show much greater resistance to extinction (Goodrick, 1968). Along similar lines, Corke (1964) showed that older rats perseverated more with incorrect responses (sequencing) on a bar-pressing task than younger rats. Combining the observations of more perseveration in the face of incorrect responding and the increased resistance to extinction has led researchers to postulate that older individuals are more "rigid" in the learning situation than are other age groups (Botwinick, 1967). Other researchers, however (e.g., Jarvik & Cohen, 1973), have suggested that the smaller age differences found in studies of instrumental versus classical conditioning should simply and practically suggest that the former be used in further experimental work with the aged. For example, in the case of discrimination training with the elderly subject, the extra time needed to learn an initial discrimination may be decreased through the use of positive reinforcement contingent upon faster responding. Jarvik and Cohen (1973) found that, by giving clear instructions and utilizing operant reinforcement procedures, the traditionally observed age differences in learning and other tasks are minimized.

Age differences are often found in studies designed to measure memory as well. Age differences are often found in studies of rote learning, memory for newly learned verbal material, and the learning of incidental material (Spencer & Dorr, 1975). In serial learning and paired-associate tasks, older persons tend to respond more slowly and make more errors than younger persons. Dichotic memory studies, using material presented in the auditory mode, show that there are age-related decrements in the recall of the second list recalled but not the first. This difference is thought to be due to a lesser depth of processing (Craik, 1977). Whenever the task involves a split of attention, the elderly as a rule perform more poorly than younger subjects. This difference is less noticeable in the auditory mode of presentation. Dichoptically (visually) presented material results in a 15% decrease in visual sensory memory in the older age groups. Walsh and Thompson (1978) found that the longest interstimulus interval for recall in younger subjects (mean age = 24 years) was 289 msec while subjects with a mean age of sixty-seven years have an ISI of 248 msec. When asked to perform multiple recall functions or when reorganization is demanded, the auditory mode appears superior to the visual mode of presentation for older subjects (Taub, 1975).

In other tasks thought to involve primary memory processes (Craik, 1977) there are few differences in the accuracy of response though the speed of response may be slower with age (Anders & Fozard, 1973). This equality in the accuracy of recall does disappear, however, when the elderly subject is presented with multiple sources of input or must reorganize the input in order to increase output accuracy. For example, a study by Kousler and Kleim (1978) using tests of multiple-item recognition learning showed that elderly subjects give more attention to irrelevant stimuli, thus less time to the processing of relevant information. However, the elderly subjects recalled less incorrect words when subsequently tested (Kousler & Kleim, 1978). Interestingly, age differences in the amount of irrelevant stimuli attended to were present only when four-item alternatives were presented and not when the correct choice was presented with only one other item. This finding is in conflict with a study by Waugh, Thomas, and Fozard (1978) which showed, in an error-free recall paradigm, that retrieval time decrements occurred in lexical, primary, and secondary memory stores regardless of the number of stimulus-response alternatives provided in subjects over the age of sixty.

Using Craik's (1977) terminology, studies measuring secondary memory processing show more age deficits. Secondary memory is thought to involve retrieval from a store in which rehearsal is not taking place. Rehearsal is experimentally prohibited by the addition of competing information, or by longer intervals between acquisition and testing. Bruning, Holzbauer, and Kimberlin (1975) found age differences on tasks designed to tap processes of long-term memory, and Smith (1975), using interference, found that males in the sixty- to eighty-year age range tended to show more memory decrements in long-term capacity than in earlier stages of processing. The fact that such decrements occur, however, is less important than the reason for such decrements. In this regard it is important to note that free recall tasks produce the most drastic age differences. This suggests that when unaided, retrieval cue effectiveness is somehow impaired and that it is poor retrieval, not trace decay or a failure in storage that produces the observed memory differences.

Of extreme clinical significance is the elderly person's ability to remember temporally remote events. Accurate assessment and intervention depend upon the accumulation of accurate facts regarding historical events in the client's life. Researchers (e.g., Bahrick, Bahrick, & Wittlinger, 1975) have consistently shown that caution is warranted in the acceptance of such personal history as given by the aged person himself. There do appear to be significant age deficits in the retention of remote events, as well.

Age-related decreases in memory performance *are* present in the elderly population. However, modifications of traditional experimental procedures often result in a decrease in these age differences. When time to respond on many of these memory tasks is increased, elderly persons' correct responses increase more than those of younger subjects (Arenberg, 1965, 1973). Also, with an increase in the anticipation interval, older subjects show a larger gain in the number of items recalled than younger subjects (Monge & Hultsch, 1971). Age-related differences have even been reported to disappear totally when self-pacing methods are used (Canestrari, 1963). When instructed to sort materials in a free recall task, performance improves over that with a nonsorting procedure (Hulicka & Weiss,

1965). When elderly subjects are given prior rehearsal with super-ordinate terms before a free recall task, no age differences are found in terms of the number of items accurately recalled (Laurence, 1967). Laurence found that by increasing the number of cues by providing the subjects with category names which are present during the recall phase, there are no significant differences between older and younger age groups.

Hulicka and Grossman (1967) found that the elderly use less pictorial mediation than the young. When instructed to mediate in this manner the elderly benefited more, in terms of items recalled, than younger subjects. Their performance on a paired-associate task was still poorer but the margin of this difference was reduced. The increase in performance by elderly subjects after instruction in the use of mediational strategies, coupled with the fact that the elderly tend to have difficulty in shifting tasks without step-by-step direc-tions (Botwinick, 1973), indicates that some of the commonly ob-served age-related decrements may be reduced through the use of instructions prior to the task. Along with instructions, training in organized strategies, decreases in the amount of interference, the use of additional cues, increases in the meaningfulness of the items used (Howell, 1972), increases in the number of concrete versus abstract items (Witte & Freund, 1976) and slower or self-paced learning or recall phases (Canestrari, 1963; Doty & Doty, 1964), may also par-tially remove the significant age differences on memory tasks.

One unfortunate consequence of the interpretation of the data from learning and memory studies has been the inference of a trait present in elderly persons which is not present in younger people. The frequency of omission errors, the tendency to repeat erroneous choices, and the longer shift durations have combined to lead some researchers to postulate that the elderly are somehow more cautious or rigid than younger persons. It has been pointed out that the elderly tend to avoid risk situations (when avoidance is an alternative) more than their younger counterparts (Botwinick, 1973). Also, intellectual performance may suffer due to this observed cautiousness. Birkhill and Schaie (1975) compared 88 elderly subjects (mean age = 73 years) either in a high-risk or low-risk group taking the Primary Mental Abilities Test. Those subjects receiving instructions intended to instill high risk did significantly poorer on the verbal meaning, space, and reasoning measures of the PMAT than those in the low-risk group when an option to respond or not was given. This finding agrees with that of Botwinick's (1966, 1969). Using a hierarchical risk-taking survey of the type which had previously revealed age differences but by not giving the option to completely avoid making a decision, it was found that older subjects are *not* more cautious than younger subjects. These findings suggest that optimum test performance would be elicited if prior instructions included the statement that there is no penalty for responding incorrectly while there would be a penalty for omitting answers (Birkhill & Schaie, 1975). Furthermore, Bry and Nawas (1969) found that this so-called rigidity is a learned phenomenon and is associated with reinforcement, intervals between reinforcement in the subject's history, and contemporary events. These findings suggest that optimum responding on tests of intellectual ability could be brought about by the use of reinforcement and cognitive training in cognitive tasks, increasing self-assurance in a risk-taking situation, and by reducing anxiety for making errors of commission (Birkhill & Schaie, 1975).

## INTELLECTUAL BEHAVIOR

It has long been thought that performance on intelligence tests decreases significantly after a certain age. This decrease in the intelligence quotient was thought to indicate progressive impairment of intellectual functioning. Even with the early returns from longitudinal studies this age difference, although much less significant, still reliably appeared. Breaking the intelligence test score down into its component parts, however, yields some rather interesting and important information. Generally, subtests which make up the Verbal IQ score yield approximately the same scores throughout chronological age while subtests designed to tap performance intelligence show a decrease in scores with age. This decrease in the Performance IQ score is often sufficient to produce the overall deficit in the general or Full Scale IQ score.

In a study of fifty-six individuals given the Wechsler Adult Intelligence Scale (WAIS) by Birren and others (1963), the following average scores were obtained. In a younger group, 10 was the average scaled score on all subtests. The Verbal scaled IQ score was 60 and the Performance scaled score was 50 with an overall IQ score of 110. For the elderly subjects, scores were above 8 on the Comprehension, Information, Vocabulary, and Arithmetic subtests; above 7 on the Similarities, Digit Span, and Picture Completion subtests; slightly above a scaled score of 6 on the Object Assembly and Picture Arrangement subtests; and averaged 3 on the Digit Symbol subtest. The Verbal scaled score was 49, the Performance scaled score was 28.5 and the Full Scale IQ score was 77.33. These figures tend to agree with the majority of intelligence assessment studies (e.g., Schaie & Strother, 1968; Spencer & Dorr, 1975) which show that while verbal capabilities are approximately the same in the various age groups tested, subtests which are designed to measure psychomotor speed, spatial integration, and perceptual-manipulative skills decline after the age of sixty. Looking at a more molecular level, it is not surprising to find an elderly person performing more poorly than a younger person on the various tasks which make up the total Performance IQ score. These tasks are typically timed, and require fine eye-hand coordination and some degree of manual dexterity. Since fine motor control, reaction time, and time perception are at less than optimum levels in the elderly, the poorer performance is understandable. To say that general intellectual ability declines with age is not understandable.

It must be stressed that difficulties abound in the assessment of intellectual functioning in the elderly population. For example, these tests typically contain very few items which have ecological validity for the elderly person. Consider the behavioral explanation for the surprisingly high relationship between early childhood scores on intelligence tests and later school performance. The strength of this relationship is based upon the commonality of the two situations (test and class) and the responses required in those situations. Certainly, the items on these tests contain material which requires the same skills as successful school performance, hence the fairly high correlation. In senescence, no such commonality is present between the test responses and the stimuli frequently encountered, nor the skills necessary for adequate performance. Therefore, the validity of such tests is questionable. Also, the typical testing situation shares stimulus elements in common with the laboratory setting. These stimulus complexes involve artificiality and stress and insufficient instructions which may differentially affect the performance of an aged individual.

In general, it appears that a clinician should not preclude treatment with an elderly person based upon an assumption that intellectual functioning naturally declines. And the clinician should not shy away from therapies which attempt to restructure cognitive problem-solving abilities in the elderly or which contain a high degree of verbal instructions or self-monitoring. In other words, modification in the sophistication of a therapeutic program should be based on variables other than chronological age.

## HIGHER ORDER PROCESSING

Several researchers have explored the functioning of elderly persons on more complex learning tasks such as concept formation and problem solving. If early theories about the general decline in cognitive processes with aging are true, this decline should be most noticeable in more complex tasks than performance on intelligence tasks or memory tests. Indeed, more significant age differences are found on more complex tests such as those involving the description of similarities, logical reasoning, analogy completion, tasks of analysis and synthesis, and inventiveness (Spencer & Dorr, 1978, p. 78). The most important observation regarding this area is that the provision of more time to respond on these tasks *does not* eliminate the age differences in performance, though special techniques such as the teaching of strategies (Goulet, 1972), use of more concrete stimulus items (Arenberg, 1973), and encouraging the overt verbalization of strategies during testing (Crovitz, 1966) may reduce age differences slightly.

The poorer performance on these types of tasks is usually hypothesized as being due to a deficit in the ability to organize complex material, deficits in short-term memory, lack of ability to make fine discriminations, and the tendency to withhold responses (errors of omission) when not sure of the correctness of the initial response. It has also been reported (Arenberg, 1973) that during testing the aged make more inquiries than younger subjects and that these inquiries are of a less information-gathering nature than those of younger subjects. This abundance of noninformative inquiries is thought to be due to a defect in the ability to form general sets or in the extraction of general rules (Welford & Birren, 1965). It is as though the elderly individual generally has a more difficult time seeing the general strategy and shifting strategies which is necessary for accurate and rapid problem solution.

The almost universal observation of more cautious responding, particularly with highly complex tasks, has led Botwinick (1967, p. 158) to postulate that cautiousness is a reasonable adaptive strategy. Instead of postulating rigidity or cognitive defect, it may be preferable to consider this rather typical behavior on the part of the elderly as a natural consequence of the self-monitoring process which tells the elderly individual that the senses, the perceptions, the memory, and the manipulative dexterity are no longer as infallible as they may have once been. To take more time to withhold responding until the level of confidence increases would then be an understandable, though relatively detrimental, strategy.

It follows that if it is overcautiousness rather than endogenous decline that lies behind the normal age differences generally observed, and if this cautiousness could be modified, then performance on the typical experimental tasks should be more similar between age groups. Coleman (1963) has provided optimism for the first link in this corrective chain. Through training with positive reinforcement, Coleman modified "rigidity," in an elderly sample, which is defined here as the inability to shift attention among concepts in a problem-solving task. "Rigidity," then, is an operant behavior which can be modified by manipulation of consequences. Since previously cited findings have shown that, at least with most tasks, special attention to motivational and instructional factors prior to experimentation reduces age-related decrements, the picture is complete. Modification of overcautiousness, perhaps through increased familiarity and learned attack or organizational strategies may lead to a "reclamation of lost abilities."

## BIOCHEMICAL AND PHYSIOLOGICAL CHANGES

The changes which accompany the aging process at the biochemical and physiological level serve, in part, to answer the proximal (as opposed to the ultimate) question as to why we age. The main difficulty in the interpretation of age-related behavior is the high incidence of changes which are only *correlated* with the progression of chronological time. Senescence is marked by an increase in physical disorders and the presence of these symptoms has often confused the analysis of "normal" aging.

At the biochemical level, there appear to be no significant consistent changes in hematological values in the elderly (Birren et al., 1963). There is a decrease in serum albumin levels due to a change in body protein metabolism and the ability of the liver to synthesize the serum albumin at the same rates. There also appears to be less adrenocorticotropic hormone, less radio-isotopic iodine uptake, more fat, and more necrocytosis among the elderly. The most important changes at this level are the decreases in cerebral blood flow and arterial oxygen saturation. Birren et al. (1963) caution that these decreases are not due to aging per se, but rather due to arteriosclerosis which causes cerebral circulatory insufficiency and anoxia. This deficiency in circulation, in turn, causes a reduction in cerebral metabolic rate and accelerated cell loss.

At the level of the connective tissues, there are decreases in the quality of tissue produced due to decreases in acid mucopolysaccharides, extractable collagen, and in the replacement rates of elastin (Sinex, 1975, pp. 25–26). These age-related changes are responsible for the stereotypical changes observed readily in elderly persons, such as loss of skin and muscle tone and wrinkling.

There is a high correlation between aging and lipofuscin accumulation. The relationship is so strong that these fatty grains are commonly referred to as the age pigment (Bondareff, 1977; Sekhon & Maxwell, 1974). These grains gather postsynaptically and impair synaptic transmission, which may account to a small degree for the slower reaction times found in the elderly (Jarvik & Cohen, 1973, p. 251). The most important clinical finding regarding lipofuscin accumulation is that abnormally high lipofuscin content is also found in patients with Huntington's chorea and chronic alcoholism. It is interesting to note that both conditions, particularly in their latter stages, resemble "dementia." No causal relationship, however, has yet been determined.

Decrements in the functioning of the ANS may well be the most clinically important change related to aging. Adaptation, the process of self-regulation in response to endogenous and exogenous change, may well be the single most relevant area of deterioration brought about by, or at least correlated with, the passage of years. Adaptation is regulated by the activity of the ANS with consequences for both cognitive and overt-behavioral involvement. As Frolkis (1977, p. 178) states,

> It is through the ANS that primarily age-related changes occurring in nervous centers may induce essential shifts in metabolism and structure and function of organs in an aging organism. Furthermore, changes in the ANS and vegetative functions per se may lead to disruption of the activities of the centers and to changes in the behavior of an aged person.

Autonomic nervous system changes include decreases in the number of fast conducting fibers and the small phasic fibers thought to be responsible for nervous activity (Jarvik & Cohen, 1973). Also present are decrements in the quality of function in the hypothalamus, sympathetic and parasympathetic systems, and in responses to the release of certain hormonal transmitters and vascular receptors (Frolkis, 1977). These changes have long been recognized as important for psychopharmacological management but should also suggest age-related differences in the nature of emotional and behavioral response and the ability to respond adequately to change.

In the central nervous system many elderly, particularly those labeled as dementia patients, show evidence of senile plaques in the hippocampus and frontal cortex, neurofibrillary tangles and degeneration, abnormal microtubules, large vacuoles, and the presence of the age pigment (lipofuscin) in the brain (Sinex, 1975). Neuroaxonal dystrophy of the nucleus gracilis is also commonly found among the aged (Berry, 1975, p. 61). Changes in the neuropil including loss of dendritic spines, the shrinking of dendritic branches, and decreases in extracellular space have recently been discovered (Wisniewski & Terry, 1976). Reactive synaptogenesis, the formation of new cellular connections after cell death, has been found in young and old rats (NIH, 1979) but the appropriateness of such compensatory growth is more variable in older organisms, sometimes leading to inappropriate behavior. In general, there is a reduction in overall brain weight such that by the age of 75, the brain weighs 8% less than at age 30 (Leaf, 1973). Other changes in central processing include a reduction in the number of functioning cells in selective areas, an increase in the random activity of cells, and longer after-effects of cerebral activity in the elderly brain (Welford & Birren, 1965). Another finding of particular clinical importance is the significant decrease in the transport capacity of norepinephrine and dopamine in the aging rat (Bondareff, Narotzky, & Routtenberg, 1971). Decreases in these essential transmitter substances have been implicated in a variety of psychopathologies including depression and schizophrenic behavior.

Electroencephalogram recordings, which should indicate any gross central process changes accompanying aging, show moderate electrocortical changes in activity. Usually about 81% of the normal elderly persons tested show normal patterns on the EEG. Though this finding at first appears reassuring, what is considered normal EEG patterns for persons over the age of 65 is not the same as for the young. When similar criteria are utilized for all age groups, only 66% of the elderly tested are within "normal" limits (Birren et al., 1963). Generally there is a 1-cycle slowing of the EEG in advanced age, with an increase in 7- to 8-cycle activity and a major decrease in the 11- to 12-cycle range. Wang and Busse (1969) found that alpha averaged 10.2 to 10.5 cycles per second in their young sample and 8.0 cycles per second in their aged sample, indicating a slowing of alpha activity. Surwillo (1968), viewing the EEG as a master timing mechanism, feels that this slowing accounts for the increases in response latencies, the greater variability in response speed, and the greater amount of time spent with complex stimulus configurations typically used in experimental studies with the aged. However, Thompson (1976) and Obrist, Busse, Eisdorfer, and Kleemeier (1962) find correlations between this slower EEG configuration and cognitive processes only in moderately to severely mentally or physically impaired elderly subjects.

In summary, the elderly show slight deficits in cognitive functioning and a slowing in processing which often presents as slower response speed and cautiousness not observed in younger subjects. The observed deficits are partially reduced through the modification of traditional procedures or by the teaching of special tactics prior to the required performance. Also, as it has been pointed out by Birren

(1970), cognitive and physiological processes are probably more related to the health status of the subject than to the subject's age. However, there are age differences consistent and significant enough to suggest the use of different normalization standards when presented with problematic behavior in an older adult. These age differences in processing and function suggest two other important points. First, changes in processing at any level should be considered as possible etiological factors or antecedent events which may lead to psychopathological response. Decrements in central and peripheral processing, receptors, coding, and response may directly produce inappropriate behavior as in the development of hallucinations, paranoid behavior, and depression secondary to reduced sensory input. Also, the responses to these age-related changes may be inappropriate and may, in turn, lead to further maladaptive behavior. For example, losses in the quality of memory function may be easily recognized by the elderly individual but may be attributed to overall deterioration, physical disease, or psychiatric involvement rather than the normal, universal, and partially remediable problem that it is. Anxiety and depression may easily result from this misattribution.

Second, given the slight decrements which do occur, the clinician should be ready to modify the interview, assessment devices, instructions, homework assignments, session length, and the process of therapy itself when the client is elderly. This is not to suggest the need for a highly specialized methodological or theoretical approach to the treatment of elderly individuals (i.e., clinical gerontology), but rather that one should address the elderly client as any other client. That is, one should attempt to maximize the probability that a successful outcome to the intervention will occur. Such an attempt necessitates the careful recognition of the strengths and deficits which that client brings to the treatment setting.

## IMPLICATIONS FOR A MODEL OF AGING

The results of the experimental studies using elderly subjects has led to a variety of hypotheses as to the major source of the age differences as well as to more molar theories designed to explain the behavioral observations. Slowing and loss of optimal functioning has been thought to be primarily due to dysfunction of sensory mechanisms, synaptic delay, slowing in the peripheral impulse transmission, slowing of the central processing mechanism, etc. Others have addressed the question of aging by hypothesizing less appropriate cellular response to stress (Sinex, 1975, p. 35), distorted or absent cellular information, injury to DNA, loss of reserve capacities, cell death, an increase in nonfunctional cells, increased errors in cell division (mutation), a decrease in the efficiency of the autoimmune system, or a change in the collagen molecular structure (cross-linkage theory) (Strehler, 1961; Verwoerdt, 1976). Theories presented to account for the behavioral observations have also been less than useful. The disengagement and activity models do not consistently fit behavioral data. Some individuals are satisfied to withdraw on reaching senescence, others simply switch sources of high activity in order to be satisfied. These theories do not effectively address the ultimate (evolutionary) reason for man's aging, nor do they go a long way in explaining the variability in behavior which often accompanies aging. More importantly, neither the biological nor the sociological theories aid in the process of clinical behavior assessment and therapy. There is a higher frequency of psychological disorders and other behavioral inadequacies including withdrawal and mild depression which can only be attacked from a wider perspective. In the next two chapters an account of growing old is presented which attempts to explain the findings of the experimental research in relation to the frequently observed inappropriate behavior. It is hoped that this new model will successfully address several questions, some of which include why persons age, why some of the elderly population behave in inappropriate and maladaptive ways, and, perhaps more importantly, why many elderly individuals do not.

# 2
# The Compensatory Model: Explaining Age-related Differences

The nature of the experimental findings designed to evaluate normal aging suggests several things. First, the quality of performance of a variety of systems (structure and function) is poorer, as measured on experimental tasks, among elderly subjects than younger subjects. Second, responses on these tasks suggest that part of these age differences are due to factors not inherent in these system changes. Third, these "artifactually" induced differences may be reduced or eliminated through modifications of the experimental procedure or the behavior of the elderly subjects.

These conclusions, based upon experimental observations, suggest a possible approach to aid understanding of the behavior of the elderly in nonlaboratory settings. It is also hoped that the abnormal behavior frequently exhibited in this population may become more understandable and a general therapeutic approach apparent. Before discussing this new attempt to synthesize the observations, two long-standing models are described.

## MODELS OF AGING

There are two popular theories to explain the psychological phenomena associated with growing old. These theories do not address the issues of the age-related changes discussed in the previous chapter directly, nor do they consider the biological or evolutionary pressures for senescence. The first theory is the *disengagement theory* which states that elderly individuals choose to withdraw from society's rigors and demands if they wish to maintain a sound psychological equilibrium. The healthy and satisfied elderly person disengages him/herself successfully from the pressures and responsibility inherent in the previous interaction with society. This theory emphasizes a passive acceptance of reduced functionality and importance on the part of the elderly individual. According to this theory, the elderly individual who resists a change in status, activity level, and previously held aspirations, will become troubled, depressed, and frustrated. However, it appears that passive withdrawal from society is not a universal motif, and is related to the educational, social, and physical status of the elderly person involved (Botwinick, 1973). In other words, some elderly individuals do withdraw from the previous demands, others do not, and the difference may be related to factors which suggest adaptive competency.

The second major model of aging developed in opposition to the disengagement model states that successful aging occurs only when the previously active individual can find other channels for his or her activity after the age of 65. The elderly person must seek other avenues of activity in order to remain psychologically healthy since society has eliminated the previously available options. The person who is thwarted in this endeavor will respond in a depressed, anxious, or otherwise inappropriate manner. Certainly, this *activity model*, as with the disengagement model, does not explain a large percentage of elderly persons' behavior. It is probably true that a previously active individual would be more likely to pursue an active retirement, but many such active persons would like to slow down and enjoy the fruits of their prior labors. Again, it appears that it is not sufficient to predict the behavior of an individual in the advanced years by his/her interaction with society. Behavior in later years is less a function of the relationship with the dictates of society and whether or not society reinforces high or low activity levels and more the ability of the elderly individual to deal with the myriad changes, both internal and external, which correlate with the aging process. In other words, predictions of behavior and the topography of behavior in the senescent stage of life are more dependent upon the endogenous changes which have taken place and the resources available to compensate for these changes. However, this relationship is not meant to be an oversimplification of the standard law of behavioral predictability. Behaviorally oriented clinicians are fond of saying something to the effect of, "The best predictor of future behavior is past behavior." While this is true (barring physical intrusion), it is a less than helpful guide in predicting the behavior due to developmental change. The assumption behind such a cliché is that there are certain commonalities in the stimulus situation at one point for an individual, and a temporally distant point in time even if the only common element is the person. This is true in part since the person not only responds with some consistency, but also emits constant stimuli which tend to elicit similar responses from others. This assumption of continuity is strained, however, when not only are the stimuli strikingly different, but also the endogenous changes which naturally occur, so the person as stimulus-generator has changed to a significant degree. Therefore, any predictions regarding behavior in the elder years based upon behavior in earlier years is made less reliable. One needs to assess the internal changes as well as the quality of adaptability in order to make any accurate statements regarding an individual's behavior in the later years. The two previously mentioned models do not take these important variables into consideration. The compensatory model is an attempt to eliminate this error.

## The Compensatory Model

The nature of the responding on experimental tasks by the elderly is typically that of a slowing and a hesitancy to commit responses. It may be convenient to view this general cautiousness and withdrawal not as result of vast physiological, sensory, or cognitive deterioration directly, but rather as a response to the natural changes which accompany aging. As Schwartz and Peterson (1979, p. 21) state:

Multiple losses (or decrements) accumulating through the middle and later years are seen as working against the maintenance of self-esteem. According to this notion, then, successful aging depends on structuring or modifying the environment in such ways as to compensate the elderly for losses—physical, social, economic, psychological. Given appropriate compensation, the senescent individual can continue to function quite effectively and with great satisfaction.

Due to the increasing limitations placed on the system, the individual no longer seeks arousal but rather seeks less arousal, actively conserving energy by preferring simplicity. With a decrease in sensory acuity, an individual may come to avoid certain situations, repeat more familiar behavior, and require more structure in unstructured situations. As Dibner (1975, p. 89) states, the often observed age differences on performance tasks may be due to "adaptation to lessened resources" rather than irreversible structural changes. This decrease in resources is coupled with a natural decline in adaptive competence (Timiras, 1972) and adaptation is the basis of the compensatory model of aging. Viewing the data in this manner not only eliminates much of the pessimism regarding modification of the behavior of the elderly, it also suggests that increasing incentives for more flexible responding and the teaching of successful coping strategies and skills may eliminate the commonly observed negative (nonconstructive) behavior. In this model, the elderly person is seen as trying to adapt to changes in function of a physical nature as well as to changes in the social environment (Havighurst, 1968, p. 69), decreases in social reinforcement (Back & Gergen, 1966), and differences in the responsiveness to stress by the autonomic nervous system (Thompson & Marsh, 1973). Since behavior of the elderly often occurs in the presence of less environmental information, it is not surprising that one observes "rigidity," the withholding of responses, less risk taking, and response times longer than a slowing in reaction time would predict. Given this analysis, Lawton and Nahemow (1973, p. 634) state:

On this basis, one would expect to find perceptual and cognitive mechanisms being used to reduce the complexity of the environment, so that objects and situations come to be of manipulable proportions. There is, of course, an inevitable loss of fineness of discrimination and the possibility of maladaptive behavior inherent in such minimization.

By viewing the behavior of the elderly in experimental settings in terms of *adaptation to the natural changes occurring* in aging, the data become understandable.

The attempt to conserve resources leads to the utilization of more primitive cognitive styles: field dependence, leveling, repression, external control, homeostasis seeking, and preference for simplicity. Field dependence and an external perceived locus of control relieve the individual of the task of searching for appropriate behavioral modes within himself. Leveling, repression, routinization, and simplistic cognition have the effect of reducing the number of external cues to be discriminated. Thus, stability is achieved through cognitive styles that reduce the internal and external demands on the individual for complex response. (Lawton & Nahemow, 1973, pp. 657–658)

The physical and cognitive resources that the individual brings into the senescent period determine the limits of adaptive ability (Lieberman, 1975). Therefore, an individual with competent adaptive skills earlier in life should show less maladaptive behavior in the later years. The relationship between past and future behavior, then, is strong *because of the generalizability of adaptive strategies.* With adequate adaptive skills an elderly person may not show the effects of any physical and psychological decline even in stressful situations. It should be noted, however, that even with competent compensatory skills, evidence of a lowered resistance to environmental change suggests an inability to compensate totally (Timiras, 1972).

The importance of adaptive behavior in early life is obvious. Man increases the probability of his survival up to the reproductive age with adaptive behavior and successful responses to environmental change (Burnet, 1974, p. 11). As Strehler (1962) states, senescence is defined as ". . . changes which occur generally in the postreproductive period and which result in a decreased survival capacity on the part of the individual organism" (p. 11). Generally, then, the deterioration which normally accompanies aging not only reduces adaptive proficiency, but also requires the use of adaptive behavior more than at any other time in order to compensate for such decreases in proficiency. The elderly person, then, is in a double bind. He or she must compensate for the loss of adaptive ability *and* for the decrease in sensory acuity, memory deficits, and slower response times. He or she must also compensate for the environmental and social changes which are imposed. With improper preparation or a history of inappropriate response to change and stress this compensatory behavior takes the form of slowing down, taking less risks, making more errors of omission, and the withdrawal from social interactions and other situations which may reveal decrements in functioning. It is reasonable to continue this analysis further by hypothesizing that more maladaptive responses may occur if the internal changes are major, the stress intense, or the coping resources particularly deficient. This may result in depressive reactions, paranoid thinking, hypochondriasis, and more total withdrawal.

It would be extremely naive to argue that all of the psychological disorders which are found disproportionately in the geriatric population are a result of inappropriate adaptation to multiple changes. Certainly, many of the age-related correlative behavioral abnormalities observed in the elderly are results of organic processes and accelerated tissue loss. However, even with organic etiology, the compensatory model may be applied. Since organic dysfunction further limits the ability to adapt to stress and to other organic deficits the overt behavior which is presented by these individuals is a function not only of organicity but also of negative response to that organicity. The fact that many elderly individuals can function adequately for many years with organic deterioration while others do not, suggests that the problematic behavior is due, at least in part, to functional determinants. Basically, these functional determinants involve the capacity to function in the face of internal and external pressures. In situations which demand sophisticated cognitive manipulations or complex skills, even those individuals with superior coping strategies who have chronic organic involvement begin to exhibit behavior uncharacteristic of previous functioning and that which is less appropriate than individuals without such organic impairment. When the demands are relatively uncomplicated it may be that the behavioral correlates of cerebral loss never become problematic enough to meet the attention of family members or mental health professionals.

This compensatory model, then, handles the observed behavioral differences exhibited by the elderly, particularly the troublesome variability encountered in this age group. What is yet to be explained in order to make this model complete is a molecular mechanism for aging. Though there is great variability in the individual response to aging and, thus, the behavioral manifestations, the physiological changes are universal. This universality suggests genetic influence.

It now appears that the process of aging is indeed based upon genetic determinants, perhaps placing the source of the changes which accompany aging within the genotype. Microbiologist Hayflick (1968, p. 37) promotes this view.

. . . the death of cells resulting in the demise of specific tissues is a normal, programmed event in the development of multicellular animals. By the same reasoning we can surmise that the aging and finite lifetime of normal cells constitute a programmed mechanism that sets an overall limit on an organism's length of life. This would suggest that, even if we were able to checkmate all the incidental causes of human aging, human beings would inevitably still succumb to the ultimate failure of the normal cells to divide or function.

This normal process of a programmed life-span may occur in DNA, with its source in the property of proteins. Either an inherent degeneration of the process of cell division and repair or a pile-up of errors is responsible for aging and cell death. The error catastrophe hypothesis states that errors or mutations in the key enzymes take place, leading to a pile-up of errors (Strehler, 1962, p. 111). Inefficient functioning and vulnerability to disease develops and these, in turn, determine life-span.

Hayflick (1977) reports the average life-span of *in vitro* cultured normal cells to be around 50 doublings. Even when the doubling process is interrupted by subzero temperature, the total number of doublings before and after the storage remains at approximately fifty. Many of the functional losses in normal human cells which precede this limit of cell division are responsible for the age-related changes frequently observed. Before the cell division ceases, the quality of the cell's function declines.

Life-span, then, is genetically determined for each species and is mediated by the genetic expression on key enzymes concerned with the replication of DNA. Any degree of error leads to error catastrophe and cell death. Errors may occur in the brain and lead to Alzheimer's or Pick's disease ("senile dementia"). Errors in the fibroblasts and epithelium result in the characteristic age changes such as wrinkles and loss of muscle tone. Somatic mutations may also lead to various neoplasia which are typically associated with aging. Along with these symptoms caused by genetic dysfunction, random or stochastic incidences may also play a role (Strehler, 1962).

The changes which occur due to the preprogramed command are changes in chemical structure. When these changes are not directed toward adaptive functioning, they are labeled as part of the aging process. Qualitative loss of function occurs naturally and can be seen in the degeneration of peripheral, autonomic, and central processing function with senescence. The reason that higher order animals, including man, tend to have longer life-spans than lower order animals may be due to the fact that human cells have evolved a more efficient system for correcting or compensating for these changes (Hayflick, 1968).

The fact that parents with long lives tend to have children with long lives is further support for a genetic basis for aging. It may be argued, of course, that external variables such as better nurturance may play a major role in this relationship. Rockstein (1958), however, found that this same relationship between length of life in parents and offspring holds with lower animals and their offspring, thus giving less equivocal support to the influence of genetic pressures. Cross-cultural observations suggest genetic contributions as well. The Vilcambians in Ecuador, the Hunza tribe in the Pakistanian Himalayas, and the Abkhazians in the Caucasus Mountains are replete with extremely old persons. Although a variety of factors may play a role in this differential longevity, such as diet, decreased temperature, and the relative absence of stress, the most striking similarity among these peoples is their geographic inaccessibility. This physical isolation tends to promote genetic isolation and a protection of genetic programming. Genetic isolation allows for the perpetuation of a process favorable for increased longevity, for instance, error-free key enzymes in the gammaglobulin and cholesterol, from one generation to another. If it is somehow advantageous to live a long time past the point of being reproductively successful in these tribes, increased longevity should continue to flourish since outside influences of "inferior" genetic messages are minimized.

The physiological changes evidenced in the elderly population which cause the behavioral changes often observed both in the experimental settings and in more naturalistic settings can now be seen as resulting from natural programmed aging. The total schema representing the compensatory model then is presented as Figure 2-1. Intrinsic mutagenesis brought about by qualitative deficiencies secondary to a finite number of cell divisions leads to the physical developments such as deterioration, slowing, sensory dulling, and

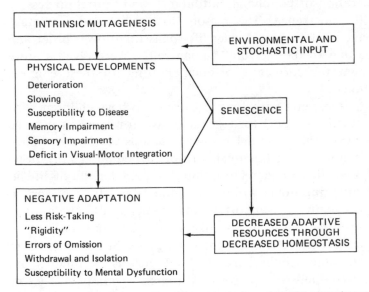

*Compensation occurs at this point and may take the form of negative adaptations unless proper strategies are utilized. The elderly person is not only compensating for decreased physical functioning, but also for a general decrement in adaptive resources. It is at this point that psychotherapeutic intervention should occur.

Figure 2-1.    The Process of Aging and the Compensatory Model.

impairment of visual-motor integration. These changes are perceived by the elderly individual and may be attributed to some disease process or significant limiting process thus resulting in behavioral adaptations, such as withdrawal and depression, often observed. Added to this inappropriate compensation for physical decrements is a lessened ability to generally adapt to change with advanced age.

## THE ULTIMATE QUESTION

In order to place a bottom line to the spiraling theorizing which has preceded, a final step in the analysis of senescent behavior should be attempted. So far only proximal issues have been addressed. These answers include the normal age-related behavioral decrements due to normal age-related physical decrements which are due, in turn, to preprogrammed aging whose locus is in the genetic process. Still, the ultimate question which remains is "Why is there a period of senescence at all?" This question is far more complex than one might imagine. The following discussion which attempts to address this question offers little practical guidance or clinical significance. It is included only as an exercise for those who either relish infinite regression, demand closure, or simply enjoy escaping applied matters for a time.

### Sociobiology and Aging

When discussing the increased longevity of certain isolated tribes we mentioned the genetic isolation which permits the continuance of genotypes which promote long lives and relatively good health. The presence of such genotypes suggests that increased longevity is "favored" in the first place. However, one is hard pressed to explain why an individual lives beyond the termination of reproductive potential. Why is there a developmental period such as senescence at all? Indeed, most organisms have little or no time between loss of potency and death (Timiras, 1972). However, in humans, females in particular, there can be many years between loss of fertility and death through cell dysfunction. The passing of cultural mores and counseling (Sinnott, 1977), while important, ignores the question of *individual* benefits. This nonfunctional period seems to place the mechanism of reproductive success in jeopardy.

Sociobiological theory encompasses a possible solution to this problem without sacrificing the "selfish" nature of evolution. This solution involves *inclusive fitness* through *kin selection*. In eusocial insects (e.g., ants, termites) and other organisms, asexual members of a group expend energy and sacrifice their own reproductive potential for closely related members of the same species or group. A closer look at these species suggests an explanation consistent with the demands of natural selection which may be used as a model for senescence.

Almost all species which contain nonreproductive castes are haplo-diploid. Males possess one set of genes, the females two sets. There-fore, the distribution of communal genes leads to the unconventional situation where female workers are more closely related to their sisters (three-quarter communality) than to their own potential off-spring (one-half communality) (Hamilton, 1964). Thus, an evolu-tionarily sound reason exists for this "altruistic" behavior which retains the essentials of natural selection while handling the existence of nonreproductive individuals. Female workers maximize their inclusive fitness by helping to maximize the reproductive potential of their more closely related sisters.

Kin selection may be applied to human behavior as well, as Barash (1977) suggests. Relatedness among humans and other diploid species varies from one half (parents and their offspring and full siblings) to one quarter for uncles and aunts with their nieces/ nephews and between grandparents and their grandchildren. Other factors enter into the likelihood of an altruistic act occurring such as recipient need, the reproductive potential of the recipient, the level of risk, and the consequences of the act on the direct reproduc-tive potential of the benefactor. This latter variable is of particular relevance since, all things being equal, grandparenting behavior should be highly probable because the reproductive potential of the benefactor (grandparent) is minimal. Inclusive fitness, which includes both the production of offspring *and* the representation of genetic communality through relatives, allows for a logical explanation for the senescent period. Evidently, grandparenting is of such sufficient importance in increasing inclusive fitness that it outweighs the lack of direct reproductivity inherent in advanced years. Therefore, the inclusive fitness of an individual is enhanced and the "selfishness" of the evolutionary process is left intact. The elderly individual who cannot contribute directly to the gene pool can *only* work to insure that those shared genes in relatives are protected. This protection and nurturance behavior is, in essence, the only behavioral option left for the elderly.

Senescence, then, should be marked by close physical proximity with other generations. This closeness insures that the mechanism for kin selection works. Other necessary criteria, which the kin selection explanation shares with the theory of reciprocal altruism, are a long life-span for the recipient and the presence of easily recognizable individuals who have a high probability of returning the "favor." The first criterion would be true for the grandparent-grandchild interaction. Also, there should be no difficulty among humans in the recognition of individuals with a high probability of returning the altruistic act since verbal communication, written records, and phenotypic similarities enhance the possibility of detecting closely related individuals from the background population. The main drawback of the reciprocity explanation alone is the rather short time remaining in the altruist's life. There must be adequate time between the altruistic act and the altruist's death to insure a high enough probability of a return on the initial investment to outweigh the costs of that act. The altruistic gene would not be continued if the chance for a return on the investment was lower than the cost of the behavior. Therefore, it seems more likely that pure kin selection and not reciprocal altruism is responsible for the senescent period of life.

Assuming that these theoretical arguments regarding mechanisms are valid, we are left with an almost impossible set of empirical tests. Direct manipulation of antecedent conditions is, of course, obviated with human subjects, but cross-cultural differences in familial patterns may help to support the ideas presented above. It is interesting to note that in the "long-lived" cultures of the world, such as the Abkhasians and the Hunzukut tribe in the Pakistanian Himalayas, the elderly individual is *elevated* in status. His or her guidance is revered and respected rather than reduced as in most civilized cultures. It may be that this reverence for age plays a causative role in the increased life-span. The additional longevity may be selected for in the same way that aunting behavior may be favored.

Given the enhancement of the elderly's role in these cultures and the geographically and genetically isolated nature of their populations, it is tempting to explain their relatively longer and healthier lives in terms of natural selection. The molecular mechanism derived from genetic isolation is undertermined but may involve the passage of relatively error-free key enzymes in the gammaglobulin and cholesterol from one generation to another. Thus, we can see the relationship between proximal explanations (genetic isolation and error-free enzymes) and the ultimate explanation (continued or increased involvement in the daily activities by the aging individual). Further observations are needed to support the contention that these long-lived tribal members are contributing directly to the enhancement of the survival of younger, related individuals. The teaching of survival skills itself may be sufficient to increase the likelihood of the prereproductive or reproductive kin's surviving to bear offspring.

Direct clinical implications suggested by this sociobiological view are few. Except for the use of elderly individuals as mediators in the treatment of childhood disorders, the enhancement of the elderly in this culture, in accordance with the foregoing hypotheses, is not to be accomplished solely through individual psychotherapy. It may be, however, that a partial explanation of the disproportionate frequency of depression among the elderly may be due to unsatisfied demands indirectly brought about by natural selection.

The preceding discussion is an attempt to complete the chain of theorization. It is a digression, however, from the major task at hand, that of describing effective therapeutic intervention. It must be stressed before addressing clinical issues that the two problematic areas emphasized in the model, that of response to change and strategies of response, involves behavior. As such, they are lawful and amenable to prediction and modification. In other words, the behavioral deficits and excesses which result from inappropriate response to age-related phenomena can be comfortably analyzed within a behavioral framework.

Arguments will be made in the final chapter for a behavioral approach to geriatric psychology. For now, two points should be sufficient as an introduction. First, though aging is correlated with qualitative changes in behavior, the relationship between behavior and its antecedents and consequences is no different. A behavioral or functional analysis is generally helpful in the acquisition of information regardless of one's theoretical or practical orientation. Second, the reliance on empirically generated information, operational definitions, and the lack of regard for hidden dynamisms, all of which are correlated with the behavioral label, are behaviors which are needed to attack a relatively new problem area. When present they are helpful in reducing the probability of making Type I (seeing something that is not there) and Type II (overlooking a pertinent relationship) errors.

The next chapter will attempt to introduce general behavioral techniques with regard to the implications which follow from the compensatory model. We approach these techniques with the view that active modification of inappropriate behavior in the senescent period of life is not only possible, but is also preferable to the behavior which is a consequence of more traditional views.

# 3
# The Compensatory Model and Behavior

The compensatory model of aging describes possible antecedents and responses which occur frequently with advanced years. The most important emphasis of this model involves the description of inappropriate behavior as resulting from inappropriate adaptation to senescent changes or, more directly, to the changes themselves. Therefore, the outwardly observable behavior problems can be seen as end products (except for discrete organic processes and resultant behavior change)[1] of this less than satisfactory adaptation process.

Two related factors, which stem both from the experimental and clinical observations of elderly individuals' behavior and the compensatory model, suggest several strategies for approaching problems of senescent behavior. These factors are the lowered competency of the elderly and the consequences of reduced input on the behavior of the elderly.

## MODIFICATION OF THE RESPONSE

The first factor that the clinician should consider is the possibly lowered competencies of their elderly clients. This deficit in response efficiency may be due to any of the factors explored in Chapter 1

---

[1] Even in the relatively straightforward case of discrete organic dysfunction causing behavior change, nonorganic factors may, and usually do, contribute to the topography of the problematic behavior.

(i.e., reduced homeostatic competency, reduced autonomic nervous system efficiency, generally reduced educational history, etc.). Regardless of the source of reduced responsivity, response facilitation is an important goal. Consideration of qualitative differences, due to age, at the level of response efficacy, leads to two general goals for the therapist. Such decrements lead to the *building of competency* with such techniques as problem-solving training and self-instructional training, and to the *training of appropriate responses in lieu of naturally occurring anxiety or withdrawal.* These inappropriate responses may preclude the utilization of competency skills which have been exhibited in the past history of the individual. This latter goal may be effected through anxiety-reduction methods such as relaxation training, stress management, or stress-inoculation training, or through selective reinforcement of nonwithdrawn behavior. We will review the basic premises and procedures which represent these two approaches before discussing applications designed to increase stimulus control.

## Training Increased Competency

Moos (1974) stresses the importance of teaching, not responses to specific stimuli, but rather more generalized coping processes.

> The goals of identifying adaptation and preventing maladaptation both imply still another reason for assessment—that is, to effect changes in adaptive behavior and in coping processes. Attempts to decrease maladaptive behavior are legion, and corresponding attempts to increase the probability of adaptive behavior, though not quite as frequent, are rapidly becoming more popular. On the other hand, direct attempts to alter individual coping processes experimentally are relatively rare thus far. The implications of the development of successful techniques to change individual coping styles could be enormous, especially if these styles actually do underlie extensive behavioral domains. (p. 336)

Generally, research generated by both nonbehavioral and behavioral researchers on the teaching of coping strategies has shown that, not only do coping strategies and problem-solving tactics change after adequate training in these methods, but specific behaviors, such as depression and frustration, change as a consequence. Fairly recently, under the rubric of cognitive behavior modification, two well-tested therapeutic approaches have emerged, self-instructional training and problem-solving training.

**Self-instructional Training.** The reader is referred to the first three chapters in Meichenbaum's (1977) book for the history and detailed utilization of self-instructional methodology. The basic assumption underlying this treatment approach is that the modification of the covert behavior (self-talk) through initially external manipulation, will lead to the modification of overt behavior (performance on some task or a decrease in inappropriate behavior). What is actually being taught is a *procedure* or a *strategy* which, it is assumed, can be used successfully even when the nature of the problem, task, or situation changes. For instance, instead of training the relaxation response as a counterconditioned response which is incompatible with phobic anxiety and hoping that this newly acquired relaxation behavior will be applied to other anxiety-producing situations, the therapist is actively attempting to program-in generalization of treatment effects by modifying the one element which is common in both situations—the individual's self-talk.

Self-instructional training usually involves several stages. First, the client is asked to analyze the problematic situation or task and look for the negative statements which he or she is using during the course of confrontation. Then, more positive self-statements are taught the client and he or she rehearses these outloud and then covertly. Oftentimes, modeling is used, whereby the therapist confronts the situation or task and verbalizes constructive self-instructions, completes the chain of behaviors required and then the therapist reinforces him- or herself with reinforcing statements. Then, the client is asked to practice the behavior overtly and then covertly, making sure to utilize the self-reinforcement statements at the completion of the entire chain. Reinforcement on completion increases the likelihood that a similar, positive chain of behavior will occur when confronted with other demands to perform.

As will be seen in Chapter 5, negative covert behavior in the form of derogatory self-statements or less than useful guides to perform are frequent problems in the elderly population. The common negative perceptions of aging are shared by the elderly population and are frequently present to prevent completion of a desired set of responses. Also, the changes which are correlated with aging often result in self-labeling which, in turn, results in an elderly person's giving up before completion of a task. Failure to complete even small chains of responses may result, then, in the complete avoidance of any active confrontation in the future. This results in the behavior often observed as withdrawal, errors of omission, or rigidity. It is quite predictable, in a behavioral light, that behavior which is followed by unpleasant consequences, such as failure or lack of positive reinforcement, will soon disappear entirely. Alternatively, experiences of completion of a task with resultant reinforcement, whether it be due to completion alone or some more contrived reinforcement, should lead to the occurrence of the entire chain of behavior in subsequent situations. Looking back at the results of the experimental findings it becomes apparent that the reduction in traditional age differences on experimental tasks when reinforcement is provided, strategies are taught, or instructions are made explicit, may be due to the same processes inherent in self-instructional training. The application of self-instructional training to specific behavior problems in the elderly will be illustrated in Chapter 8.

**Problem-solving Training.** Behaviorally oriented psychologists have lately recognized that competency in the ability to solve difficult problems is an important target for modification. Goldfried and D'Zurilla (1969) describe the need for the assessment of behavioral competency and the steps involved in such evaluation. First, the individual's ability to conduct a situational analysis is evaluated. Definition of the problem situation is imperative before solutions can be tendered. Then, response enumeration occurs in which all responses to these situations are listed. The individual then must judge the adequacy of each response alternative in a process termed response evaluation. The two final stages of response competency involve measuring the instrumentation of the selected solutions and calculation of validity and reliability of such measures. D'Zurilla and Goldfried (1971) believe that such a process fits well into the overall paradigm of behavior therapy (p. 109).

It should now be clear that the goals of problem solving and behavior modification are one and the same, namely, to stimulate
behavior which is likely to produce positive consequences, that is,
positive reinforcement, and avoid negative consequences, that is,
negative reinforcement. Training in problem solving, therefore,
may be viewed as one of several possible behavior modification
techniques for facilitating effective behavior.

Goldfried and Goldfried (1975, p. 104) have developed a five-stage
therapeutic program which includes: general orientation, operational
definition of the situation and formulation of goals and conflicts,
generation of alternative strategies, decision-making (selection of the
best strategy and tactics), and verification of effectiveness.

The first stage indicated by Goldfried and Goldfried (1975),
general orientation, is based upon the assumption that an individual's
set and attitudes can affect the way they face a situation. During this
stage, the treatment rationale is presented and the factors which may
contribute to the occurrence of difficult situations are discussed.
This recognition of problematic situations is accompanied by stress-
ing the negative results of responding automatically, without thinking, when faced with a challenging situation. Common situations in
daily life in which problems may arise are brought out and examples
of common problems are explored. The client is taught to use the
unpleasant feelings which often accompany the presentation of
problematic events as cues or signals to explore the causes of these
feelings. During the second stage, problem definition and formulation, the client is taught to define in operational terms all aspects of
the problematic situation and to classify the elements of the situation as to their relevancy or irrelevancy. Goals and issues are identified and possible conflicts between goals are discussed.

The next stage is the generation of alternatives, in which possible
solutions to the problem are generated through the method of brain-
storming. This generation involves stating as many alternative solutions as possible without critically evaluating their likelihood of
success. No judgments are made during this stage since it is assumed
that a deferment in judgment ultimately leads to more effective
problem solving and that the generation of alternatives in large
quantities will lead to the best final decision (Parnes, 1967). When all

possible alternatives are specified, the decision-making stage begins. Johnson, Parrett, and Stratton (1968) have suggested that subjects may require certain guidelines in the selection of the most appropriate strategy and tactics to pursue as well as in the estimation of the subjective utility of a decision. During this stage the consequences of the various alternatives are explored after a rough screening which attempts to eliminate highly unlikely or impossible alternative strategies from consideration. The personal, social, short-term, and long-term consequences of a particular action are explored and ranked according to the likelihood of occurrence and the likelihood of success. When the best alternative or alternatives are carefully selected, the client returns to the generation-of-alternatives-stage to select the best tactics for the implementation of these strategies. Estimates as to the valence of the consequences of each tactic are then made. D'Zurilla and Goldfried (1971) summarize this stage (p. 119):

> In the case of the selection of the best strategy to pursue in a problematic situation, the value of the strategy is judged against its likelihood of effectively resolving the major issues or conflicts. In the case of the evaluation of specific means of implementing the strategy selected, the effectiveness with which the strategy is implemented is used in estimating its value.

The final stage of problem-solving training involves testing of the solution(s) which were scored the highest during the decision-making stage. After the course of action has been chosen, the client tries out this solution either imaginally or in an actual situation. This process is described by D'Zurilla and Goldfried (1971, p. 120).

> In order to deal with a problematic situation at more than just a hypothetical level, the individual must carry out the selected course of action, either in the life situation or by role-playing the situation, observe the various consequences of his actions, and test or match this outcome against his expected outcome. If the match is satisfactory, the problem-solving process can be terminated. If the individual finds the match to be unsatisfactory, however, he continues to "operate" (i.e., returning to the problem

definition and formulation, generation of alternatives, and/or decision making), repeating this procedure until a satisfactory match is finally achieved.

If the problematic situation is handled effectively, the results of this success serve to reinforce the sequence of problem-solving behavior and thus, increases the probability of the entire chain of behavior occurring in the future.

The relevance of this situational problem-solving approach depends upon the assumptions that psychological difficulties such as depression, can be caused or aggravated by inefficient coping skills and that these coping skills can be taught in such a manner as to be effective in a variety of problematic situations (Goldfried & Davison, 1976). These authors suggest that problem-solving training may be particularly appropriate with patients who have recently or soon will be experiencing role transition. This would include hospitalized and incarcerated individuals. The suggestion here is that the self-control, which is believed to accrue after problem-solving training, will be helpful in dealing with newly acquired independence and responsibility after release. It follows that problem-solving training might also prove to be helpful when the transition between institution and community is reversed. In a situation where dependence is the norm and previously successful strategies and tactics are inadequate or insufficient the individual may require clearly defined and systematic training in adaptive problem-solving. One such a situation is entrance into an institution for the physical and/or psychological care of the aged. Typically, the transition from home to institution is abrupt and the role contrast is striking. This transition, coupled with the changes which accompany "normal" aging can lead to maladaptive responses such as depression and suspiciousness.

The training of efficient problem-solving techniques then, can be seen as fitting into the compensatory model as an attempt to either restore or establish more functional responses. An approach which involves cognitive modification rather than direct environmental manipulation is important particularly in those cases where the condition of the client, the nature of the problem, or the composition of the environment renders external change impractical. Given the nature of the traditional settings in which the elderly often are located and the severity of many of the correlated physical ailments, "internal" modifications which lead to more effective adaptation to existent situations may be the *only* possible course. However, in many cases the adequate response may be present but is suppressed or overridden by inappropriate responding to such an extent that such competency building is initially prohibited. In these cases the inappropriate responses which are obviating appropriate response must be modified first.

## Reducing Inappropriate Responses

During assessment of response deficits, behavior therapists have found it necessary to distinguish between skills deficits and skills suppression. Skill deficit suggests an inadequacy of response or set of responses primarily due to the lack of previous similar stimulus-response-reinforcement experience. The present context is less relevent, therefore, than the individual's learning history. Skills suppression, on the other hand, is defined in light of the immediate environmental situation and the presence of a competing response or set of responses. These competing responses are usually less adaptive than the suppressed skill and among the elderly, generally take the form of anxiety, depression, chronic complaints, and/or suspiciousness.

Four general approaches which are designed to reduce these immediately critical responses are muscular relaxation training, systematic desensitization, stress-inoculation training, and the shaping of increasing participation in ongoing activities. The first three approaches are aimed at the reduction of anxiety, while the last, the use of contingent positive reinforcement for interacting with the environment is an aid in the reduction of depression and withdrawal. A reduction in depression, theoretically (See Chapter 5), should lead to a decrease in two other common inappropriate responses, suspiciousness and chronic multiple somatic complaints.

**Relaxation Training.** The training of a relaxation response was traditionally a precursor to passage through the hierarchy in systematic desensitization. Wolpe (1969) included such training so as to provide the client with a conveniently available response which the client could emit, which was incompatible with the previous inappropriate responses of anxiety and avoidance. When confronted with an anxiety producing situation or stimulus, the client is instructed to utilize his or her newly acquired relaxation response which had been counterconditioned to the previously anxiety-producing situation instead of inappropriate arousal. Recent research has cast a dubious light on the necessity for formal relaxation training in the process of systematic desensitization, though it has persisted as the most popular substitute response for anxiety. Relaxation alone has been used in the treatment of insomnia and generalized anxiety and as one component in a variety of other behavioral techniques such as stress-inoculation training and flooding relief.

It is important to note that many correlated physical changes present in the elderly prevent the use of complete formal muscular relaxation training. Loss of muscle tone, inability to tense properly, contractures, and old fractures make such a rigorous process impossible. However, more cognitive forms of relaxation training, or training which does not involve the usual tension-relaxation sequence may be useful in cases of extreme agitation. Relaxation as a response, and the process of relaxation as a skill may reduce anxiety sufficiently to allow the therapist to institute other forms of therapy, such as those involving response-competency building.

**Systematic Desensitization.**   The most widely used and researched treatment of a behavioral nature is systematic desensitization. The main assumption behind systematic desensitization is that the anxiety which is currently resulting from contact with a particular idea or item will be eliminated if an incompatible response is paired continually with that idea or item.

Traditionally, the therapist and the client first develop a hierarchy in ascending order of anxiety (increasing the temporal or spatial proximity of a phobic or anxiety-producing stimulus or situation). Then, muscular relaxation is trained or some other strategy is taught, such as the use of positive, approach-enhancing coping statements. Then, the client is slowly taken from one step to another, pausing only when anxiety becomes intense. He or she is instructed to use relaxation or image the coping statement when the anxiety begins to become unbearable. The ultimate goal of such gradual ascension through the hierarchy is to enable the client to come face-to-face with the previously anxiety-producing stimulus in the absence of the usual responses (anxiety, arousal, and/or avoidance). Though the entire process may and usually is conducted imaginally, real stimuli or situations, whenever practical, may also be used and the approach of the client or the movement of the stimulus item is then varied until contact or appropriate performance is obtained.

Though phobias do exist in the elderly population, most of the use of systematic desensitization typically conducted with this age group involves gradual introduction to more generalized themes. In other words, the typical analogues found in the literature involving snakes, spiders, and public speaking are replaced by more amorphous and less easily defined fears such as fear of institutionalization, fear of being alone, fear of rejection, and the fear of loss or dysfunction of a body system or part.

In the cases mentioned above, the anxiety which precludes the utilization of any competent strategies which may be available is typically due to misinformation or insufficient information about what to expect. In these cases, it is often observed that only the initial steps of exposure to the *in vivo* or *in vitro* situation need to be accompanied by an alternative response such as relaxation or positive coping statements. Therefore, two or three sessions devoted to such training is not advantageous since informal practice is often enough for the client to approach the final steps of the hierarchy with no overt signs of anxiety or escape. Also, the clinician dealing with elderly clients should consider shortening the session length and using age-relevant coping statements ("I will not let my failing eyesight prevent me exploring this new facility") to increase the probability of treatment success.

**Stress Inoculation Training.** Stress inoculation training, as explained by Meichenbaum (1973) and Meichenbaum and Turk (1976), is a procedure which assumes that the clients internal dialogue is an important factor in anxiety reactions and that the modification of cognitions is as important as the modification of overt behavior. If cognitive events are viewed as ". . . specific sets of self-statements and/or self-instructions which the client could be trained to alter," the possibility for modification becomes apparent (Meichenbaum,

1973, pp. 6–7). Stress inoculation training is similar to other coping skills methods such as self-instructional training and problem-solving training in that the strategies of approach to a problematic situation are targeted for change on the assumption that modifications of such strategies will lead to changes in behavior.

In stress inoculation training, the client is first instructed as to the nature of anxiety reactions within a cognitive-behavioral framework. Second, the client is asked to rehearse coping behaviors, and last, he or she is provided with an opportunity to practice the constructive coping skills that have been learned in the presence of the stressful stimulus. This exposure phase differentiates stress inoculation training from self-instructional training (Meichenbaum, 1977).

The educational phase provides the client with a cognitive framework to explain his or her stress reaction. The treatment rationale is presented, and the number of sessions and scheduling are decided upon. The rehearsal phase may include a relaxation training period though this component may be eliminated with no change in efficacy. Relaxation and regular breathing is encouraged, but muscle relaxation training is not mandatory.

The client is then asked to report his or her own negative self-statements which are usually present during the anxiety-producing situation. Then, incompatible self-statements are suggested, with the client being the originator of the statements to be used. These positive statements involve four areas: preparation for a stressor, confronting the stressor, facing the possibility of being overwhelmed by the stressor, and reinforcing oneself for successfully coping in the situation. These positive statements are rehearsed by the subject aloud and then covertly.

After proficiency has been established, the subject is instructed to practice these new skills in the presence of the stressor. The purpose of this practice is that the presentation of the initial stress-producing stimulus will force the exercise of the new coping skills without the threat of catastrophic results. New attack strategies are exhibited without resulting in the previous responses of anxiety or avoidance.

Stress inoculation training and related coping skills procedures have been found to be effective in dealing with a variety of problems including test anxiety (Meichenbaum, 1972; Wine, 1970), nonassertiveness (Glass, Gottman, & Shmurak, 1976), the control of anger

(Novaco, 1975), preoperative stress (Langer, Janis, & Wolfer, 1975), and ischemic pain (pain due to artery constriction through thermal stimulation) (Turk, 1978). In the application of stress-inoculation training to anxiety with many elderly clients it may be most beneficial to choose, or reinforce the client's choice of coping statements emphasizing slightly different components than typically used with younger clients. Statements which are more concrete ("If I move my walker slowly and carefully I will not fall" vs. "There is no reason to be afraid of falling") and which contain references to past positive coping behavior ("I didn't let those steps bother me when I fractured my hip last Fall" vs. "I know I can handle those steps if I try hard enough") tend to be more effective.

Stress-inoculation training, then, can be seen as another method designed to reduce maladaptive responses prior to the programming of adaptive response(s). Since the procedure involves the teaching of a skill (recognizing anxiety cues, covertly rehearsing positive coping statements, and appropriate self-reinforcement) this approach also can be seen as a method to build response competency. This second aspect occurs naturally after the maladaptive behavior has been eliminated in the presenting problematic situation. Therefore, successful stress-inoculation training may be seen as the end-point in therapeutic intervention (except for booster sessions when necessary for maintenance). One further point should be mentioned which encourages the use of stress-inoculation training with elderly clients. The present generation of elderly individuals tend to assimilate the common-sense value of "talking-oneself-out-of-difficulties" and the "power-of-positive-thinking." This generation, probably more than future cohorts of elderly persons, have been reinforced for dealing with problems as they occur independently of external influences (particularly mental health professionals). Therefore, initial acceptance of the procedures is easily obtained and future implementation of the procedures is made more likely since it appears to the client that his or her behavior is once again under personal control. It is impossible to underestimate the value of increased self-control for an elderly individual.

**Shaping of Increasing Interactions With the Environment.** Depression is the most frequently encountered maladaptive response of the elderly. Unlike depression occurring in younger age groups, the therapist should not be content with a high remittance rate since without active intervention of some kind, geriatric depression not only fails to remit but usually worsens. Though many approaches have proven successful (e.g., problem-solving training) the most widely used and researched is the gradual shaping of increasing participation in activities through contingent positive reinforcement. Gradual approximations to the desired goal usually require fairly continuous reinforcement in the early stages (out-of-bed, out-of-room behavior) but more intermittently thereafter. This is probably due to the intrinsic reinforcement properties of the more advanced target behaviors at the terminal end of the chain.

The main assumption of such an approach is that an increase in activity level corresponds to decreases in depressed behavior. However, one must not be content to accept increases in activity level alone as representative of reduction in depression since, by most definitions of depression, a low activity level is just one criterion for labeling an individual's behavior as depressed. Monitoring other indices of depression such as appetite, sleeping patterns, and feelings of sadness and despair, must be included in order to verify this treatment approach.

Once the withdrawn behavior with concomitant suspiciousness and somatic complaints has been reduced, competent response building, if necessary, may begin.

Important age-related modifications of this common procedure include the use of age-relevant reinforcers (e.g., pictures of a young Bette Davis or Lionel Barrymore, roll-your-own cigarettes, and snuff) and age-relevant activities (e.g., needlepoint, bean snapping, and visits by young people). We are often surprised when a program involving the standard reinforcers (i.e., candy and packaged cigarettes) fails to work, but in retrospect, we should expect such null results.

So far in this chapter we have discussed some general methods to increase the efficiency of responding either through direct response modification or the modification of competing, inappropriate responses. Many other techniques, particularly in the second category, could have been included. In most cases, the age of the client does not necessitate large procedural changes in any of these techniques (e.g., flooding, flooding relief, modeling). However, regardless of the nature of the population served, behavior therapy has long maintained a tradition of idiosyncratic treatment development. Procedural modifications, when necessary, are limited only by the common sense and creativity of the therapist.

## REDUCED INPUT AND REDUCED STIMULUS CONTROL

In addition to difficulties in the nature of the response, experimental and clinical observations also show difficulties at the stimulus or input level. Though it may appear that our discussion is not in the logical sequence as suggested by functional analysis, problems involving input deficiencies are addressed secondly for an important reason. In most routine practice with elderly clients in most treatment settings, age-related input differences are not relevant. It is only the smaller population of geriatric clients who present greater dysfunction who necessitate consideration of problems of stimulus control. This smaller population is usually residing in long-term care, nursing, or geriatric facilities. By considering problems in this area secondarily, it is also hoped that the clinician will be helped to realize that such a population is not representative of the elderly cohort.

Most of the treatment approaches mentioned above as response-facilitating require some degree of cognitive facility. Unfortunately, a small but nevertheless significant number of behavioral problems are exhibited by geriatric clients who do not possess such ability, at least initially. Much of these individuals' inappropriate behavior is a consequence of reduced input. This reduction in the quality and quantity of information may stem from inadequate information in the environment, altered sensory receptivity, limited central processing, or a combination of these factors (See Figure 3–1). Deficits in these areas suggest the use of "supernormal" stimulus control, special attention to the types of reinforcement, and the magnification of conditioning components.

### Supernormal Stimulus Control

A large percentage of the inappropriate behavior witnessed in the traditional settings in which the elderly reside is not in and of itself

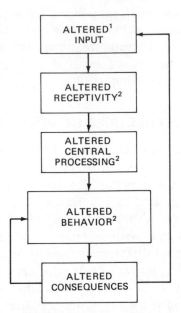

<small>[1]</small> Altered may be defined as decreased, modified, or changed in quality.
<small>[2]</small> Correlated disease processes may compound alterations at these levels.

**Figure 3–1.   Potential Sources of Alteration of Behavior in Senescence.**

inappropriate. When the behavior is taken from the context in which it is creating negative responses in others and placed in any number of different contexts the behavior loses its inappropriateness. For example, when we observe an elderly patient in a nursing home urinating or masturbating in the main lobby, most observers would label that behavior as abnormal. In some cases, such observations would agree with common misperceptions of the elderly. However, if such behavior occurred in the appropriate bathroom and in the appropriate receptacle, even if observed by these same individuals, the labels of abnormal or perverted are less likely to be used. In this case, *the behavior itself should not be the target of change but rather the behavior-in-its-present-context should be changed.* This problem, of course, is not confined to the elderly though it appears that, in this population, improper behavioral control by the usual stimuli is most frequent. Due to the sensory and cognitive changes which frequently are present, particularly in chronic organic loss, the elderly person's behavior often appears to be under no external control at all.

There is another reason for targeting stimulus control as well. If an inappropriate behavior has continued for a long period of time or if the functioning level of the client is very low, it is often the case that the topography of the behavior may not be modifiable. This leads to intervention techniques directed toward bringing such behavior into more reasonable situational control.

When attempting to develop appropriate stimulus control over a behavior exhibited by an individual who, for whatever reason, does not attend to ordinary cues (i.e., commodes, their own bed, ash trays), atypical or unnatural stimuli must be utilized. These artificially designed stimuli are most effective when they incorporate magnified stimulus properties. Since visual cues are most readily used and have been the cues most often responded to in earlier years, supernormal visual cues are valuable in establishing or re-establishing appropriate stimulus control. Large, vividly colored cues may be placed in the environment where the frequency of behavior is to be increased or decreased and then faded into smaller, less "supernormal" artificial cues. The ultimate goal is the complete removal of the artificial stimulus with no behavioral relapse.[2] A further step is suggested by Agras, Kazdin, and Wilson (1979, p. 130).

In addition, behavior change programs should be designed to increase the individual's independence and competence as rapidly as possible so that external control of behavior by the therapeutic regime can be reduced quickly and ultimately terminated. A considerable amount of laboratory research provides potential guidelines for facilitating diverse self-control efforts. After participants adopt new patterns of behavior, the next phase in the program may require direct training in self-reinforcement. This is achieved by gradually transferring evaluation of performance from the therapist to the client. Rewards can then be made contingent not only on the occurrence of desired behavior but also on accurate self-evaluation of performance.

[2]During the fading process it is wise to keep in mind that, due to decreases in acuity, the final stages in stimulus shrinking may not be perceived. Instructions to focus on the smaller cue may be necessary.

Specific examples of treatment programs including elements of supernormal stimulus control and self-reinforcement will be described in Chapters 7 and 8.

## Idiopathic Reinforcement

Age-related changes as well as cohort characteristics often make it necessary to depart from the usual schedules and sources of reinforcement. The nature of the level of functioning should dictate the former concern rather than age, per se. The types of reinforcement which are effective, however, do change to a certain extent with age. For example, the cultural, economic, and historical backgrounds of geriatric clients often result in certain reinforcers being favored over others. Often these biases are not the same as those held by the designer of the behavioral program. Even the well-designed and usually comprehensive reinforcement surveys neglect possibly potent reinforcers for this age group. In clinical practice, visitation, conversations about past events or locales, access to previously popular music, and engagement in practices of earlier times such as husking, needlepoint, or wood carving are often chosen by the elderly client.

## Magnification of Conditioning Variables

As discussed above, common sense dictates special consideration in the use of discriminative stimuli and reinforcers in the operant conditioning paradigm with most elderly clients. Decreased acuity across sensory modalities also demands the use of more intense conditioned and unconditioned stimuli as well (classical conditioning paradigm). In shaping procedures, louder auditory stimuli and brighter visual stimuli should be employed with the elderly in order to meet the criteria of an adequate stimulus. In aversive methods, shocks, unpleasant odors, and noxious tones must usually be more intense than those used with individuals who present no sensory dysfunction. It should also be remembered that the process of classical conditioning may require more time with elderly clients.

This chapter has included discussions of behavioral methods used in the treatment of problems associated with aging. These problems may occur due to the direct result of age-related changes, or, more frequently, to inappropriate responses to these changes (excess dysfunction). More specific assessment and therapeutic considerations in behavioral geriatrics follow. First, however, etiologies of behavior change not typically addressed in behavioral literature are introduced. The nature of senescent behavior dictates such a focus.

# 4
# Biophysical Etiology and Endogenous Stimuli

Behavior therapists have long been effective in the analysis and treatment of functional disorders and the nonorganic components of interactive (organic etiology with functional consequences and visa versa) disorders. With the advent of behavioral medicine, behavioral technology has been applied to medical problems in a variety of areas such as prophylaxis (e.g., stress reduction techniques), symptom monitoring and control (e.g., hypertension), treatment compliance (e.g., drug administration), and cognitive elements (e.g., anxiety management). However, due to the philosophical bias and focus of training, awareness of the causative relationship between biophysical processes and behavior-cognitive response has not been a key component of the behaviorist's repertoire. This awareness is essential in the assessment of behavioral problems exhibited by the elderly.

Functional analysis of the presenting problem provides a convenient format for the identification of antecedent conditions, past history of the individual, the parameters of the problematic behavior (nature, frequency, intensity, and duration), and the consequences which result when the behavior occurs.[1] The shorthand formula of functional analysis is:

[1] It should be noted that "functional" has two meanings in this context. One meaning is synonymous with "nonorganic," suggesting an etiology involving conditioning or learning factors. The other meaning simply indicates an approach in which behavioral problems are analyzed as functions of contextual factors. This latter approach may be the behaviorists' major contribution to assessment.

Stimulus————Organism———— Response————Consequences
(Antecedent events)  (Past history,  (Parameters of (Reinforcement)
                     cognitive          behavior)
                     rules, and
                     physiological
                     function)

All behavior can be subjected to functional analysis though the generality of this formula is most useful for providing a guiding framework for training purposes. Nevertheless, this descriptive process is the heart of behavioral assessment and the precursor of behavioral intervention.

This analysis is certainly helpful in the assessment of geriatric problems, though a deficit exists which is of great practical importance.[2] As noted in Chapter 1, senescence is correlated with increasing risk of physical illness and imbalances of bodily systems. Some of these maladaptive states are specific only to advanced years while most appear among other age groups though not with as high a frequency. It is important to note that though age is not a valid independent variable in research nor a useful etiological variable in clinical practice, it does, however, correlate rather highly with many problematic behaviors. These organic variables play an important role in four ways:

1. Organic etiology may lead directly to, and may even present initially, as behavioral disturbances. This can be seen in the presence of paranoid delusions secondary to uncontrolled diabetes mellitus or disorientation which results from generalized cortical atrophy.
2. Physical illnesses and debilities almost always occur concomitantly with psychological difficulties such as when the lack of mobility secondary to a cerebrovascular accident is accompanied by depression.
3. Psychological problems may present as physical complaints

---

[2]This deficit lies, not within the S–O–R–C model itself but rather in the variable descriptions as typically presented in behavioral texts. Also, inappropriate behavior which is assessed by a behavioral therapist is usually viewed as a sample of behavior, not as a sign of underlying pathology. This bias may also be detrimental.

which are reinforced by the attention of health professionals and significant others. This is frequently seen in depressed elderly patients whose depression is less noticeable than their hypochondriasis or multiple somatic complaints.

4. A third variable, psychological in nature, may cause physical symptoms which may in turn lead to further psychological involvement. An example would be inappropriate stress management leading to hypertension which then leads to anxiety in response to the hypertensive condition.

The first category, thought to lie under the jurisdiction of medically oriented therapists, is the least understood by behaviorally trained therapists and will be discussed in this chapter. The second and third categories will be dealt with in the following chapter while the final interaction between organicity and behavior is handled adequately in the literature of psychosomatics and will not be discussed here. (See, for instance, Ullmann & Krasner, Chapter 18, 1969; Wittkower & Warnes, 1977).

Organic problems may be seen as fitting within the S–O–R–C model either as endogenous stimuli or as organism variables. For example, an electrolyte imbalance may act as a *stimulus* for inappropriate overt behavior yet the process and function is definitely a part of the individual. There may be great individual differences in these processes prior to an imbalance which may predispose an individual to respond maladaptively in the absence of harsh external demands. These individual differences are, of course, subsumed under the "organism" heading. Placement within the behavioral framework is less crucial, however, than recognizing that the consideration of organic causes is necessary in geriatric psychology. In fact it is often the case, particularly if suggested in the client's medical history, that such causative factors should be eliminated *first* before proceeding with a nonorganic assessment. Whenever an obvious environmental causative factor is not readily apparent, as in relocation or death of a loved one, internal "organism" variables should be immediately explored. The establishment of endogenous involvement, however, should not preclude the assessment of environmental concomitants or the application of environmental techniques to treatment. As will be seen in Chapter 7, external modification at the stimulus and consequence points in the model may be help-ful in reducing the negative aspects of physically induced behavioral abnormalities.

Several biophysically induced behavior problems exist which are frequently observed with elderly clients. These include alterations in behavior due to psychotropic and other types of medication, acute physical conditions and imbalances, and chronic physical changes (Hughes, Myers, Smith, & Libow, 1973).

## ALTERATIONS DUE TO PSYCHOPHARMACOKINETICS

Several age-related changes result in rather idiopathic drug responses which may, in turn, cause behavioral disorders. These changes in-clude declines in organ cell population, decreased basal metabolic rate, decreased organ perfusion and efficiency, atherosclerosis, urinary retention, decreased gastric acid secretion, decreased active transport, decreased gastric motility, higher incidences of diarrhea, decreased muscle mass, reduced total body water, decreased cardiac output, lessened flexibility of cardiac reflexes, lowered plasma protein, reduced renal blood flow, changes in the sensitivity of receptors, and a reduction in overall homeostatic regulation (Chap-ron & Lawson, 1978; Masoro, 1972). Given these changes, which may be exacerbated by the presence of physical disease, the high frequency of drug-induced behavioral difficulties is not surprising. Drug therapy may cause iatrogenic effects among the elderly more often than with other age groups not only because of the aforemen-tioned physiological changes but also due to a greater variability in drug response and the higher incidence of paradoxical effects (Bassuk & Schoonover, 1977).

Table 4–1 summarizes the more frequently prescribed psycho-tropic medications, the symptoms for which they are typically pre-scribed, and the adverse behavioral manifestations which may result (Altman, Mehta, Evenson, & Sletten, 1973; Appleton, 1976; Bassuk & Schoonover, 1977; DiMascio & Sovner, 1976; Korsgaard & Skavsig, 1979; Saltzman & Shader, 1979; Whitlock & Evan, 1978). The be-havioral manifestations noted may oftentimes be masked as a more widely known complaint through the process of misattribution. This misattribution is particularly true of drug-induced akinesia mas-

## Table 4.1  Commonly Prescribed Drugs and Possible Side-effects in the Elderly.

| Medication | Typically Prescribed For | Behavioral Signs as Side-Effects |
|---|---|---|
| Anti-Parkinson | Symptoms of Parkinson's disease and pseudo-Parkinson's | Psychotic behavior |
| Digitalis | Hypertension | Hallucinations, confusion, nightmares, disorientation |
| Dilantin (toxicity) | Seizure disorders | Lethargy, confusion |
| Diuretics | Edema | Sexual disturbances, confusion |
| Antihypertensive | High blood pressure | Lethargy, depression, sexual disturbances, headache, psychotic behavior |
| Antiarrhythmics | Irregularities in heart rate | Psychotic behavior, rashes |
| Gastrointestinal | Acidity, upset, gas | Confusion |
| Steroids | Arthritis | Mania, hallucinations, delusions, emotional variability |
| Major tranquilizers<br>Phenothiazines<br>Aliphatics<br>Chlorpromazine | Combativeness, extreme agitation, hallucinations, delusions, hostility | Drowsiness, withdrawal, rigidity, akinesia,* tremor, obesity |
| Promazine<br>Piperazines<br>Fluphenazine<br>Trifluoperazine<br>Piperidines<br>Thioridazine | "<br><br><br>" | Motor restlessness (akathesia), insomnia, muscle spasms (dystonias), tongue, lip, and jaw movements (tardive dyskinesia)**<br>Sexual dysfunction, rashes |
| Butyrophenones<br>Haloperidol | As above and mania, paranoid ideations | Extrapyramidal (rigidity, tremors) |
| Thioxanthenes<br>Thiothixene | As above and severe depression | Extrapyramidal |
| Antidepressants<br>Tricyclics<br>(Desipramine, amitriptyline, nortriptyline, doxepin) | Motor retardation, hypochondriasis, poor appetite, insomnia, and self-neglect symptomatic of depression | Agitation, psychotic behavior, urinary retention, paresthesia |
| MAO-Inhibitors | Same as above | Same as above and hypertensive crises |
| Minor Tranquilizers<br>Benzodiazepines<br>Chlordiazepoxide<br>Diazepam | Anxiety, multiple somatic complaints, convulsions, insomnia, agitation | Visual hallucinations, confusion, disorientation. Psychotic behavior may follow withdrawal. |
| Oxazepam<br>Diphenylmethane<br>Hydroxyzine | | |
| Lithium Carbonate | Racing thoughts, mania, manic-depression | Anorexia, psychotic behavior |

*Mimics depression

**Mimics Huntington's chorea

querading as depression and loss of motor function and Parkinson-like tremors being labeled as anxiety. The following case is illustrative of another type of misattribution.

A sixty-three-year-old man was referred for inappropriate sexual behavior, including repetitive pelvic thrusts, frottage, and contact with female patients and staff of an inappropriate nature. It was observed, however, that this repetitive motor behavior also occurred in the presence of inanimate objects and while the client was laying down. The client had, one week prior to the emission of this behavior, been placed on haloperidol (a major tranquilizer). What initially had been thought to be a sexual aberration, despite the absence of similar behavior in the past, was actually a drug-induced dystonia (involuntary contraction). Though the client was incapable of understanding the nature of his behavior, his family was relieved to attribute it to an "external," nonvolitional cause.

The case above suggests a further problem which may follow misattribution. Side-effects (e.g., motoric, anticholinergic, etc.) are usually readily perceived by the elderly client or by family members. This is particularly true when these symptoms appear against a background of minimal external complexity, such as that found in many geriatric facilities. Reduced activity level and the bland surroundings of many institutions for the aged cause preoccupation with internally generated stimuli. These changes may then be attributed either to further declines due to aging, physical illness, or to psychological disturbances. This attribution leads to anxiety regarding this personal physical or psychological condition (Oberleder, 1966). The client may even request "something for my nerves" at this point, only adding to the problem. Or the anxiety may actually exacerbate the tremors, sexual dysfunction, or disorientation. In either case, the therapist's attention is drawn away from the pertinent link in the chain of causation. Time wasted in the assessment process or on well-intentioned but inappropriate therapeutic strategies is particularly dangerous when drug side-effects are present. Some side-effects are not only bothersome but may be irreversible if permitted to continue for even a moderate length of time. Jeste, Potkin, Sinha, Feder, and Wyatt (1979) found, for example, that after withdrawal of neuroleptic medications in twenty-one patients over fifty years of age, tardive dyskinesia (repetitive involuntary movements of the tongue and mouth such as chewing and smacking) remained in nine. The predictive factor for persistence or abatement was the length of neuroleptic treatment. Surprisingly, the greater the number of drug-free periods, the higher the chances were of persistence.

Although the prescription of psychotropic medications comes under the professional province of physicians, awareness of drug side-effects is essential for the psychologist who deals with elderly clients. Though the administration of such drugs is not a part of the behavior therapist's armament, and theoretical bias may even bring about "desired ignorance" of such therapeutics, the psychologist or other health professional should be at least cursorily familar with the major groups of drugs, their kinetics, and their undesirable consequences so as not to miss a significant number of problematic endogenous factors.

The problems which most frequently present as psychological or emotional problems that may actually be due to negative psychoactive drug side-effects include anxiety (particularly with motoric involvement such as tremors, restlessness, constant limb, trunk, or head movements), tics of the face or neck, insomnia, lethargy or lack of energy, anorexia, parasthesia, sexual dysfunction (loss of interest and/or ability to perform), dermatitis, hypochondriasis, cognitive impairment, and racing thoughts (Buchanan, 1978). Hypotension (Glassman, Bigger, Giardina, Kantor, Perel, & Davies, 1979; Rodstein & Oei, 1979) and manic behavior (Van Scheyen & Van Kammen, 1979) present less frequently. When the elderly individual complains of any of the above, assessment should include the following.

1.  Look at the medications presently being taken by the individual. Check for the presence of psychotropic medications of the types presented in Table 4-1. Determine as accurately as possible the date of initial dose, length of treatment, previous trials on that medication, and the present dosage. Narrow down the date of onset of the presenting symptom(s) and look for correspondences in time.
2.  Be particularly alert to the presence of multiple psychotropic medications since their effects are often synergistic or antag-

onistic. If the former is true, the problem may be drug related. In the latter case, it is apparent that the pharmacological treatment approach will continue to fail as a solution to the psychological problem.

3. Check with others regarding the reliability of self-administered medications. Medication which is taken above the prescribed dosages or medication irregularly consumed can cause difficulties. Ask the client to show you how many pills or capsules he/she took at the last time of consumption.

4. Familiarize yourself with the average time necessary to reach therapeutic effectiveness, potential side-effects which may occur, and the length of time a medication stays active in the tissue after termination of treatment. Widen these parameters in both directions for the elderly client since it appears that the elderly present more variability in drug response than younger clients.

5. Know the typical symptoms of withdrawal from psychoactive drugs. With certain drugs, lengths of treatment, and dosages, some rather bizarre psychotic symptomology may appear when a drug is not withdrawn at the appropriate rate. This can be seen in the following case.

> A seventy-year-old female was admitted to a nursing home with diagnoses of diabetes mellitus, cataracts, and depression. Medication on admission included rather moderate levels of meprobamate which the patient had been taking for several years. The dosage level was reduced carefully, but the patient began to exhibit visual hallucinations, anxiety, delirium, disorientation, and reported nightmares. Though the patient had had recent problems with diabetic ketosis and insulin reactions, and had confined herself to a dimly illuminated room, it was thought that the causative agent was meprobamate withdrawal not sensory deprivation or diabetic delirium. Reinstatement of the original dosage of meprobamate eliminated the problematic behavior. This case is an excellent example of judicious medical practice which nevertheless fails to predict idiosyncratic response patterns.

6.  Be alert to drug-drug interactions, drug-food interactions, or drug-disease interactions and the overt symptoms which may result with each (Hansten, 1976; McAllister, Scowden, & Stone, 1978). For example, a client may be receiving psychotropic medication at what appears to be a typical dose. If the symptoms do not abate in time and there is little question of compliance consider a drug-drug cancellation effect. For instance, oral antacids frequently taken by the elderly can inhibit the blood levels of phenothiazines (major tranquilizers). Though such cancellations of effect are not in and of themselves harmful, the lack of effectiveness of a drug regimen may encourage an increase in the amount or potency of the psychotropic which may then lead to behavioral problems if the nonpsychotropic drug is discontinued.

7.  Suspect sudden onsets corresponding to the beginning, termination, or a change in drug therapy. Since the elderly client is more likely to have been medicated for longer periods of time than younger clients, suspect lengthy medication trials or high levels of medication.

8.  Note the termination of a drug, such as an anti-Parkinson agent, which may have been prescribed to counteract neuroleptic side-effects. Parkinson-like tremors, salivation, and shuffling gait may reappear secondary to the major tranquilizer.

9.  If the client presents a problem which is commensurate statistically and physiologically with a symptom complex of drug effects, attempt to ascertain if other, commonly related symptoms are also present. Active probing is often necessary throughout the assessment process with an elderly client since errors of omission, memory deficits, and the reserved nature of this cohort make voluntary imparting of information less probable. For instance, if ejaculatory incompetence is the presenting problem for someone on an antidepressant, determine if other, anticholinergic effects are also present. These would include blurred vision, urinary retention, constipation, and/or dry mouth. The presence of two or more of these related signs is suggestive of drug-induced dysfunction.

10. A recent study by Yesavage (1979) has shown that most drug-induced problems abate within two to three days, two

weeks at the most. Therefore, a drug etiology should be ruled out if the behavior continues for a longer period than two weeks. An acute medical problem or an idiosyncratic drug response should be suspected at this point.

Knowledge of drug-caused behavior problems does not require in-depth, time-consuming submersion into the literature of psycho-tropics. When conducting therapy privately or on an outpatient basis, familiarity may be gained through the use of reference guides, formu-laries, or the Physician's Desk Reference. Clinical practice in nursing homes, long-term care facilities, and geriatric institutions can be enhanced in this regard by a close relationship with pharmacists, the physician, geriatric nursing personnel, or consulting psychiatrists.

## NONPSYCHOACTIVE DRUG-INDUCED ALTERATIONS

Almost all prescription drugs have the potential for altering physi-ology to an extent that unwanted behavioral signs may occur. With the high incidence of elderly clients receiving medication for control of medical symptoms, awareness of possible side-effects and toxicity is important to the assessment process.

Toxicity will probably manifest itself rather obviously in acute delirium and physical decompensation such that it would not present itself initially to a psychologist. More subtle manifestations, without an accompanying discrete physical onset, prove to be the most difficult etiological variable to uncover. In terms of toxicity, how-ever, it is sufficient to note that the range between therapeutic and toxic levels for most medications is narrower for elderly clients than for younger clients. Therefore, accidental drug toxicity as a cause of behavioral problems is more frequent in this population.

Table 4–1 includes the more commonly prescribed types of medi-cations for physical illness which may lead to behavioral abnormal-ities. Similar drugs and similar dosages rarely result in difficulties with other age groups, but do very frequently cause startling be-havioral problems with the elderly. The reasons for this selectivity are the same as with the psychotropic drugs. With the myriad changes which accompany the aging process, it is understandable that drugs have different effects on this population. The following cases are illustrative.

**Table 4.2   Frequent Biophysical Causes of Behavior Disturbances in the Elderly.**

| Biophysical Etiology | Immediate Cause | Behavioral Signs |
|---|---|---|
| Diabetes mellitus | Hyperglycemia and insufficient antidiuretic hormone release | Depression, agitation, paranoid ideations |
| Respiratory acidosis in emphysema, asthma, infections, pneumonia, pulmonary edema, and with sedatives | Retention of carbon dioxide secondary to hypoventilation leading to a lowered pH | Somnolence, confusion, disorientation |
| Respiratory alkalosis in hysteria, hypoxia, and with acetylsalicylic acid | Hyperventilation leading to expulsion of carbon dioxide and an increased pH | Anxiety, further hyperventilation |
| Congestive heart failure and myocardial infarction | Hypokalemia and hypoxia | Confusion, decrease in cognitive function |
| Azotemia in urinary tract infections, diabetes and with antihistamines, anticholinergics, antihypertensives, diuretics | Increases nitrogenous waste in blood | Confusion, hyperactivity, delusions |
| Neoplasm | | |
| Frontal lobe | Tissue damage | Anxiety, decreased inhibition, hallucinations |
| Temporal lobe | Tissue damage | Memory impairment, communication disorders |
| Parietal lobe | Tissue damage | Agnosia, apraxia, aphasia, hysteria |
| Occipital lobe | Tissue damage | Visual hallucinations |
| Vascular disorders as CVA, TIA, cranial arteritis, subdural hematoma | Cell loss | Emotional variability, depression |
| Infections | Water loss and electrolyte imbalances | Confusion, disorientation, depression |
| Nutritional | | |
| Pellagra | Decrease in nicotinic acid | Depression, dermatitis, cognitive impairment |
| Wernicke's and Korsakoff's | Cell loss, anoxia | Memory impairment, confabulation, ataxia, confusion |
| Endocrinopathies | | |
| Hyperthyroidism | Not specified | Hyperactivity |
| Hypothyroidism | Not specified | Depression, paranoid ideations |
| Parathyroid | Hypercalcemia | Anxiety, depression, psychotic behavior |
| Adrenal crisis | Increase in steroids | Apathy, depression, irritability, neurasthenia |

**Table 4.2** (*continued*)

| Biophysical Etiology | Immediate Cause | Behavioral Signs |
|---|---|---|
| Cushing's syndrome | Hypokalemia and hypernatremia and inappropriate ACTH level | Paranoid ideations, anxiety, apathy |
| Metabolic disorders as uremic encephalopathy | Not specified | Altered attention span, depression, asterixis, myoclonus, tremors, cognitive impairment |
| Hepatic encephalopathy | Cirrhosis of the liver | Agitation, tremors |
| Electrolyte imbalances |  |  |
| Hypokalemia | Secondary to diuretics, steroids, renal disease | Depression, anorexia, apathy, lethargy, irritability, paresthesia |
| Hyperkalemia | Renal disease | Depression, weakness, muscle spasms |
| Hypomagnesemia | Not specified | Delusions and hallucinations |
| Hypernatremia | Water loss | Cognitive impairment |
| Hyponatremia | Diuretics, CVA | Cognitive impairment |
| Hypercalcemia | Renal disease, hyperparathyroidism | Polyuria, depression, lethargy, confusion, psychotic behavior |
| Hypocalcemia | Renal failure, hypoparathyroidism | Cognitive impairment |

A seventy-one-year-old male, hospitalized for congestive heart failure and a recurrent urinary tract infection, was placed on antihypertensive medication to decrease blood pressure. One week following this regimen he began to stare for long periods of time at the walls of his room and in the hospital corridors. He became more lethargic and less responsive than on admission. A follow-up digit span test also showed a dramatic reduction in attention span and processing. The dosage of the antihypertensive medication was reduced by half and a more restricted sodium intake diet was instigated. On discharge twelve days later, the patient showed no behavioral abnormalities and his attention span returned to the previous premedication level.

A sixty-eight-year-old male with diagnoses of chronic brain syndrom (DSM–II) and seizure disorder was placed on a regimen of phenobarbitol and dilantin. A dilantin level assay was ordered for two weeks following the therapy's beginning. The patient had no problems for three months, at which time he became slovenly in appearance, walked and spoke in an intoxicated manner, wandered frequently, and looked lethargic during the day. One week later, his serum dilantin level was found to be 41 UG/ML (Normal range is 10–20 UG/ML). His dilantin was discontinued and his behavior returned to precrisis levels. In this case, as in so many, behavioral signs actually heralded biophysical abnormality.

It is a simple matter to list possible behavioral problems which may result from poor adjustment to medication. The real difficulty in the assessment process lies with the fact that the parameters of such overt signs are similar regardless of the offending medication. This is probably due to the common molecular mechanisms behind the action of such drugs. Intervention, however, is not aimed at either the overt-behavioral nor the molecular-physiological levels per se, but rather at the mediating level, the drug itself. With multiple pharmacological substances and the diverse number of potential organic and functional etiologies commonly present in the elderly, pinpointing the causative agent is difficult. In addition, given the severity of the physical condition for which the offending drug is prescribed and the limited number of alternative approaches, changing at the level of the drug itself may be undesirable. One is then left to help the elderly client cope with the negative side-effects of a medication which may be necessary for the rest of their lives.

Periodic serum levels should be obtained when the therapist suspects, either due to the rapidity of the behavior's onset or its correspondence to the initiation of a potentially offensive drug, that the presenting problem may be drug-related. Serum levels can be obtained rather easily and economically for such common culprits as lithium carbonate, dilantin, digitalis, phenobarbital, the diuretics, and steroids. These serum levels may still not be definitive since they show only possible toxic levels of drugs and would not help if the behavior is an idiosyncratic adverse reaction to the medication. When the latter is suspected, absolute dosage or time of administration may be modified and follow-up observations made for changes in behavior. It is often the case that some overt problems, such as lethargy and lack of energy can be eliminated by either lowering the amount of a drug administered or by giving the medication before retiring at night when the behavior is less bothersome. For example, this type of schedule change would alleviate the difficulties associated with drugs which commonly cause orthostatic hypotension and frequent falls. By giving such medications at night, not only is the risk of injury reduced but the patient's unsteadiness during the day may be reduced sufficiently to promote participation in ongoing activities, independence in self-care skills, and gains from other therapeutic interventions.

The usefulness of environmental manipulation techniques is undeniable and the assessment of functional variables is necessary, but it should be noted that a workable relationship with a professional who can prescribe and discontinue medication is also essential. The optimal situation in geriatric assessment is when all assessors involved in the patient's plan of care are aware of all of the possible variables, including drug effects. Valuable intervention time is wasted when perceptions on the part of and communication among professionals is rendered impossible by the narrowness of their respective approaches. An assessment team made up of a variety of disciplines is of course desirable, though this approach can be further improved upon by having team members with general enough backgrounds so that they may share viewpoints, knowledge, vocabulary, and levels of analysis.

## ACUTE PHYSICAL DISTURBANCES

One of the most controversial areas in the assessment and treatment of elderly clients is the labeling of a set of amorphous behaviors, organic mental disorders. The discussion as to the efficacy of such a designation is held until Chapter 7, but it should be kept in mind that the usefulness of the following presentation is independent of the validity of diagnostic terminology.

Acute physical disturbances may cause behavioral abnormalities in any age group. Due to some of the factors addressed earlier, however, these disturbances cause more behavioral symptomology in the elderly than in any other age group. These causes should not only be considered as a part of the assessment process, but should be foremost in the therapist's mind particularly whenever physical illness is present or has been indicated in the client's recent past. When the onset of the disruptive behavior is sudden and there is no history of past mental health intervention, one should suspect the presence of a medical etiology with this age group.

The behavioral symptoms most likely to present as a result of physical causes include anxiety, depression, sleep disturbances, changes in "personality," variability in mood, loss of concentration, disturbances of recent memory, impaired judgment, delusions, suspiciousness, and visual hallucinations (Fox, Topel, & Huckman, 1975). Concomitant with these psychological complaints may be medical symptoms including weakness, arrhythmia, changes in the pattern of urination, parathesia, headaches, and chest pain (Hall, Cruzenski, & Popkin, 1979; Steel, 1978). The foremost behavioral sign suggesting an acute physical condition with elderly clients appears to be what nursing staff, family members, or friends of the client would label as a "change in personality." This rather nebulous phrase may not contain predictive or functional value for the assessor by specifying etiology or suggesting a treatment plan, but it should be a salient cue to elicit a search for a medical, endogenous antecedent. It is often the case with elderly clients that this "change in personality" is not necessarily in a strikingly negative or inappropriate direction but rather may be a more acceptable or neutral array of behaviors that are, nonetheless, uncharacteristic of the usual pattern of response. An elderly person who perceives a problem developing endogenously may compensate behaviorally in any atypical pattern of response. The following case should serve to clarify this point.

A sixty-three-year-old female was placed in a long-term care facility primarily due to one-sided weakness secondary to an old cerebrovascular accident. She exhibited chronic complaints and utilized her *prn* medications as often as possible. Although she was capable of functioning more independently she relied heavily on the nursing staff, family members, and visitors. Rather suddenly, however, the number of requests for pain medication and aid declined significantly though no intervention had been instituted. She appeared more anxious than before, but her behavior towards others became less demanding. After two weeks, it was discovered that the patient was developing a urinary tract infection of moderate severity. After eliminating the infection the behavior returned to its previous level. On interview, the patient stated that she had "felt so bad that I thought I was going to die." This preoccupation with her physical condition, which appeared to have an organic etiology for the first time since admission, had replaced the previously bothersome and inappropriate overt behavior.

Table 4-2 presents the most frequently encountered biophysical etiologies which result in inappropriate behavioral signs (Fox, Topel, & Huckman, 1975; Libow, 1977; Steel, 1978). The importance of recognizing these common causes cannot be understated. Though the behavioral manifestations may first appear in much the same manner as the more chronic and oftentimes irreversible brain disorders they differ in one very important regard. They are easily modifiable once the etiology is determined (Libow, 1973). This differentiation may be hampered by the absence of a complete history or by unreliable reporting. The problem may be eased through referral to a physician or neurologist for appropriate testing whenever such a cause is thought to be likely. Errors or oversights in assessment may result in inappropriate institutionalization, further complication of the physical ailment, or a change in status from a temporary cognitive or behavioral dysfunction to a more permanent condition. It is a sobering exericse to consider that many of the elderly individuals in long-term care facilities and on the geriatric wards of mental institutions with current diagnoses of chronic organic mental disorders might have escaped this rather bleak existence had the acute medical cause been uncovered when symptoms first appeared. Short-term and reversible changes can and do lead to irreversible changes when left unattended. Given the disruptive nature of these acute changes, the reservedness and suspiciousness of this cohort, and the frequent lack of family contact, it is not surprising that this omission may occur with some frequency. Parker, Deibler, Feldshuh, Frosch, Laureana, and Sillen (1976) conducted a study of 116 patients, 65 years of age and older, who were referred for physical assessment while residents of a geropsychiatric facility. Forty-four of these patients were ultimately diagnosed as having acute organic brain syndrome, and twenty-three as having chronic brain syndrome. All but two of these 116 patients had at least one medical illness. Seventy-one, or 61.2% of the total, were considered to have medically caused behavior problems. Despite weaknesses in the diagnostic system and the use of medically oriented assessors in this study, this remains a highly significant figure.

It may not be clear from looking at Table 4-2 but the endogenous "bottom-line" is often an electrolyte imbalance. This is particularly true in elderly patients who are hospitalized for physical reasons. In addition, being placed in a facility for the physically ill forces the patient to cope with the novelty and sometimes sterility of a service-oriented institution. Therefore, the therapist is often faced with a recently incapacitated client who is, in addition to the illness-complex, facing unfamiliar surroundings. If, on top of these factors, hypokalemia or hyponatremia occur, depression is *very* likely to result (Stroot, Lee, & Schaper, 1975). It is clear, in this case, that the identification and elimination of the physical cause (e.g., a diuretic-induced imbalance) will not be sufficient to eliminate the depressive symptomology alone. However, accurate analysis of the depressive aspects of hospitalization and physical illness would not provide a complete picture either.

The assessment process should consider a multiplicity of contributing factors at both the molar and molecular levels of analysis. Proper treatment can not be effected if only partial assessments are conducted. The rule of thumb should be, suspect everything, then narrow down the search to find the most pertinent variables. It is the rare exception that one and only one factor is responsible for the behavior that is presented. It follows, then, that it is rare for one therapeutic approach to be sufficient to return the elderly client to premorbid levels of functioning.

When a medical agent is suspected, the therapist should actively seek a medical referral. Biomedical assays of blood and urine can be ordered by the physician which provide, among other information: levels of potassium, calcium, BUN, sodium, creatinine, BUN/creatinine ratio, protein, phosphorous, cholesterol, triglycerides, chloride, LDH, glucose, and bilirubin levels. Electroencephalograms, neurological tests, X rays, RPR (syphilis test), thyroid panels, drug screens, and liver panels might also yield valuable information.

The mental status exam is a valuable tool in assessment of acute medically caused behavioral manifestations or delirium as it is traditionally known (Eisdorfer & Cohen, 1978). A sample evaluation form is presented in Appendix A. The results of a mental status evaluation are enlightening in diagnosing acute reactions, particularly when these evaluations are conducted routinely across time to provide baseline responding from which comparisons can be made. Inappropriate behavior secondary to acute endogenous changes usually presents clearly enough on initial contact but baseline comparisons are helpful in determining the course of the disturbance. In institutions it is often valuable to administer a mental status questionnaire on admission with periodic follow-up administrations or administrations on an as-needed basis throughout the patient's stay. If the attending physician has ordered routine serum or urine assays, these may prove useful in preventing full-blown acute episodes from occurring. For assessment purposes it is important to note that, retrospectively, behavioral disturbances which have been found to result from acute physical changes in the elderly usually are suggested first by irregularities in lab values and behavior, and secondarily by clinical symptoms (i.e., nausea, vomiting, fever, dyspnea, urinary frequency, changes in bowel habits). Intervention early in this progression may prevent overt difficulties and may prevent the possibility of an acute disturbance complicating the already delicate functioning of an individual with a more chronic irreversible condition.

In assessing the problem through the use of a mental status examination, it is important to be alert for the following.

*Movement.* Observe for motor restlessness, ataxia, multifocal myoclonus (repetitive spasms), and/or constant picking at the clothes or skin.

*Speech.* Speech changes which often correlate with sudden onsets of biophysically caused behavior disorders include slurring (as in an intoxicated individual), changes in accent, and/or changes in the speed of delivery of speech. For example:

A seventy-six-year-old female, hospitalized for an old cerebrovascular accident and depression, began showing signs of slurred, thick speech, and a sudden increase in agitation. These symptoms coincided with an increase in thiothixene (a major tranquilizer with antidepressant properties) and, initially, this was thought to be the cause of the deterioration. After a physical examination revealed slight mouth drooping on one side and slight one-sided weakness over the body, it was determined that this patient had suffered a minor cerebrovascular accident once again. There was no cognitive loss indicated on a mental status exam following this stroke, though the depression present on admission had intensified. Without careful scrutiny, time would have been wasted on a purely psychotherapeutic approach or on changing the medication.

*Autonomic complaints.* Anxiety, incontinence, sweating, fever, nausea, and tachycardia are often observed or reported in conjunction with acute disorders. These signs may appear later than the cognitive or behavioral signs, but they are very significant and serve to differentiate these acutely caused problems from chronic ones.

An eighty-three-year-old female had been a resident of a long-term care facility with an admission diagnosis of cerebral thrombotic arteriosclerosis. She could carry out her own activities of daily living with some assistance and was quite independent and outgoing. Very suddenly she began to withdraw, and became confused, disoriented, combative, hallucinatory, and struck several patients and staff members. At the peak of her crisis, she had struck her roommate with a pan and collapsed. Her blood pressure at this time was 240/120, her pulse was 126, and her respiration was 54 and irregular. She was dyspneac and complained of epigastric burning. Nitrobid® resolved the crisis and after being placed in a private room, she began to recover. No further behavioral problems have been noticed one month after the crisis. Her sudden behavior change with a total course of one and one-half weeks was secondary to cerebral vascular insufficiency.

*Affect.* Intensification of inappropriate affect and heightened variability appear to almost always coincide with an acute episode. Outbursts of crying and hyperactive motor behavior often alternate with stuporous, withdrawn periods. These changes in affect are often the signs which are labeled as "personality" changes by observers since the magnitude of the changes in this area is so startling.

*Consciousness.* Responsiveness to or awareness of the immediate environment decreases during an acute episode along with attention span. Asking for a repetition of the numbers of the *WAIS* Digit Span subtest or serial sevens should expose this deficit though it may be readily apparent on interview.

*Cognition.* Recent memory appears to be affected more than remote memory during these episodes. This may be due to a difficulty in registration of input secondary to the decreased attention span. Transitions between ideas appear to be either inappropriate or nonexistent. The individual flips from one topic to another, seldom finishing any complete idea. Thinking in general appears to be less organized and associations looser.

Briefly, the most characteristic signs of a biophysically induced acute cognitive disorder are a lack of attention, motor restlessness, insomnia, decreased appetite, paranoid verbalizations, vivid hallucinations, cognitive clouding, and "personality changes." The greatest aid in differential diagnosis is the suddenness with which these behaviors appear. The most frequent causes of these abnormal responses are infectious diseases, post-trauma or postoperative states, cardiac irregularities, drug intoxification or withdrawal, postconvulsive conditions, hypoglycemia, and anemia (Adams & Victor, 1970). Elderly clients who have physical illnesses and psychological problems, as in the case of elderly psychiatric patients with diabetes, will be particularly prone to have medically caused behavior problems since they may fail to adhere to medical and dietary regimens (Wotring, 1978). A classic example which serves to show the complexity of the clinical picture is the depressed elderly diabetic whose depression may worsen for whatever reason leading to a waning of appetite. This decrease in food consumption then leads to hypoglycemia which then may lead to confusional states and a worsening of the depression. This cycle, if not broken quickly, may lead to the death of the client either through suicide or diabetic coma.

These acute biomedically induced conditions may be exacerbated by the presence of chronic cognitive changes. These chronic changes, traditionally known as "dementia," confuse the assessment picture since it is difficult to determine whether the most recent deterioration in behavior is due to the natural progression of the "dementia" or to acute changes superimposed upon a rather stable, chronic condition. Hospitalization of a client who shows dramatic decline may also further complicate the picture by adding another confounding causative factor, sensory deprivation. A decrease in sensory stimulation leads only to a worsening of the chronic condition as well as to an intensification of the disorganization brought about by the acute organic condition. Symptoms of acutely caused disorders worsen at night as do the symptoms of chronic disorders and depression among the elderly. It appears that a further reduction in the sensory stimuli which impinge upon the dysfunctional individual brings about an exaggerated deficit in response (Ernst, Beran, Safford, & Kleinhauz, 1978). With a deficit in the available external information, less appropriate responses are emitted. Given the data concerning the effects of sensory deprivation on normals it is understandable that those individuals with an already present abnormal filtering system would appear to respond inappropriately more frequently with lowered input. In point of fact, one important treatment enhancement technique in cases of behavioral disturbances due to acute medical etiology is to heighten surrounding sensory stimulation, for instance keeping the lights on in the client's bedroom continuously, until the crisis is resolved. This use of stimulation may appear counterintuitive since it would seem that bombarding an already overburdened processing system would create even more chaotic behavior, but the reverse, within reason, is the typical observation in clinical practice.

When a client is referred who has a history of chronic deterioration secondary to a progressive disease, Alzheimer's for example, but the presenting problem appears to be of sudden onset, it is probably appropriate to assume that an underlying medical disturbance or drug-related effect is present. Such superimposing of an acute reaction on top of a pre-existing chronic loss may complicate the assessment process. This is particularly true since such a combination often results in a blunting of the acute response. The behavioral signs of this "delirium" are often less intense than when an acute organic disorder is present alone. It is tempting in the assessment procedure, to hypothesize that the client's condition is simply deteriorating at a faster rate than had previously been the case. This temptation derives from the observation that in the late stages of a chronic condition such as Alzheimer's, the progression of the behavioral symptoms may actually be geometric. The staggered progression is due to the fact that different parts of the brain are atrophying at different rates leading to differential loss of function. The therapist, however, should not be satisfied that he or she is witnessing the natural progression of an irreversible process. The consequences of making an error in assessment in this regard do not lead to equally acceptable outcomes. It should be foremost in one's approach that an acute and reversible medical cause may be the origin of the most recent behavioral changes. A return to baseline functioning, no matter how regressed we may judge that level to be, is superior to making an error which would result in further decompensation when that decompensation could have been prevented.

## CHRONIC PHYSICALLY CAUSED DISTURBANCES

The organically caused problems discussed above are minor compared to those which may be subsumed under this heading. These chronic disturbances are more significant in terms of their irreversibility, debility, treatment availability, assessibility, and acceptability. This latter point, the problem of acceptability, deserves further comment. Depending upon one's approach to the correlates of aging, one will come in contact with either an abundance of clients with chronic organic mental disorders or only a few, isolated cases. Unfortunately, by the time that such cases reach most psychotherapists, degrees of freedom in the assessment process have been trimmed. What many clinicians see now, especially in long-term care facilities and on geriatric mental wards, may well be the iatrogenically induced irreversible conditions. It helps little to realize that these cases do not often result from diagnostic errors *per se* but rather from less than rigorous assessment and widely held but erroneous beliefs of years past. It cannot be denied by the sophisticated therapist that such progressively deteriorating conditions do exist at an uncomfortable rate even with rigorous and thorough evaluation. It is hoped, however, that diagnostic labels such as schizophrenia, chronic undifferentiated type; organic mental disorder; and senile dementia are less readily applied now than in the past.

### Differential Diagnosis: Chronic Versus Acute Organic Changes

There are conditions of cognitive incapacitation and behavior change which are mostly irreversible and which have widespread, global signs. These changes are highly correlated with advanced age though in no way can age be viewed as the sole causative factor. "Senile dementia" or chronic organic mental disorders are complexes of behavior which do correlate with age. When accurately and diligently labeled such chronic changes are generally progressively debilitating, show diffuse cerebral involvement, and result in less specific behavioral manifestations than is the case with acutely caused behavior change (Eisdorfer & Cohen, 1978; Reichel, 1978).

Given that an error at the level of assessment has dire consequences for the elderly client, points of difference between these chronic conditions and the more acute changes, as well as between the former and functional depression should be noted. Two factors aid in the differentiation between what has been referred to as "dementia" and "delirium." The first factor is the nature of the onset of dysfunction. In the early stages of a chronic and irreversible condition, the client shows many of the same signs as the "delirius" client, but these signs persist at the same level of intensity for a longer period of time. With "delirium," behavioral changes continue to intensify in the level of inappropriateness. With long-term changes, fine motor control (such as changes in the quality of handwriting), recent-memory impairment, multiple somatic complaints, emotional variability, and inappropriate reactions to frustration are present. Anxiety and depression may also be present. The therapist is confronted with a clinical picture similar to that of acute disorders, but the suddenness of the manifestations is less noticeable and the course less dramatic (Wells, 1976). The "changes in personality" noted with acute biophysically originating problems are not nearly so marked. In fact, it is usually the case that the client does not even perceive these subtle changes through his or her self-monitoring process. The client's family or friends, if they notice at all, usually attribute observed changes to their idea of normal aging or perhaps some external stimulus such as stress. It is relatively safe to state then that, *if a behavior becomes problematic enough to come to the attention of a physician or mental health professional, the source of that problematic behavior is probably not early chronic-organic degeneration.* Rather, the therapist should look for depression, an acutely caused organic problem, a drug response, or a chronic organic syndrome in its latter stages. Only when an ongoing assessment process is being conducted, which is only likely in an institutional setting, would the initial stages of a progressive disorder be noticed. It is usually only retrospective analysis which provides evidence for and a description of the earlier stages.

Later stages of the progressive disease yield the second differentiating factor, that of affect. After the initial signs of mild anxiety or depression, the client with a chronic disorder shows less intense affect, even to the point of indifference or denial. This period can be seen as a compensatory phase, in which the losses which are accruing are best handled by denial. Denial in this context is not the same process that psychodynamic theorists and therapists follow though the consequences of that process may be the same. Denial appears to be an adaptive compensation to reduce negative affect regarding an extremely difficult illness as perceived by the client. Through the interview or mental status evaluation it should become apparent that this strategy is present. Periodically the client who later is shown to have such an illness (either through CT scan, by the course of the deterioration itself, or by eliminating possible acute causes) will become agitated when pushed by the interviewer to make further attempts to answer a simple question or to complete a simple task. It is as if the interviewer is providing a situation which challenges the barrier of denial just enough to temporarily allow unimpeded self-monitoring to occur. For a brief time the client is faced with the gravity of his or her situation.

A second common response to persistent questioning is sudden crying. When questions are asked to gain information about the client's remote memory or the status of his or her orientation to place and time, the client may suddenly tear-up and grimace. Then, just as suddenly, the crying will stop. It is thought that questions pertaining to the past bring up uncomfortable comparisons between past capabilities and present ones and that questions which force the client to consider the present environment (such as a private office, hospital, or nursing home) lessen the client's ability to avoid acknowledging current conditions. Usually the sequence occurs so quickly that actual tearing does not occur and only the facial contortions earlier in the crying sequence are observed. It is interesting to entertain the possibility that the disorientation to time and place often seen with these clients is less a memory deficit, confusion, or some cognitive deficit, than appropriate denial.

In the final stages of progressive dysfunction, motor behavior becomes impaired, speech becomes less intelligible, unfinished sentences and neologisms occur, and the individual becomes almost totally dependent on others for their activities of daily living. The following case shows the progression of cortical atrophy.

A seventy-nine-year-old male with diagnoses of chronic brain syndrome and cerebral arteriosclerosis with senile dementia had been placed in a long-term care facility when the demands of his care became too involved for family members. On admission, the patient could follow simple commands, emit complete sentences though the content was sometimes irrelevant, was neat in appearance, and disoriented only to time. Three months later he began to leave sentences unfinished, often completing them with nonexistent words or perseverating rhymes. For example, when asked how he was doing one morning, his reply was, "I'm not to do to do to doing ninitz (sic)." On another occasion he replied to the inquiry, "Where are you going?", "I'm a going to where de where de some where over the de the rain uh spout." Two months later, disoriented to time, place, and person, this patient would often point out a nearby window to nonexistent objects.

It may be that the neologisms observed in these patients and which usually occur at the end of sentences are also attempts to cover perceived losses. By inventing a word or using a word apparently drawn at random, the patient can deny memory loss or shortened attention span.[3]

As difficult as it may be to distinguish between disorders with acute etiologies and the more chronic progressive type, the real assessment difficulty lies in the distinction between the latter and functional depression in the elderly. Again, an error at this point would be tragic since the depressed elderly patient responds well to intervention either of a pharmacological or psychotherapeutic nature. Unlike depression encountered with younger clients that

[3] Loss of contact with reality and/or denial do not take place twenty-four hours a day with these patients. The gentleman in the case above, even late in the progression of the disorder, stated with no observable precipitating stimulus, "Growing old is horrible." The sentence was complete, gramatically correct, and rather devastating.

often remits in 6–18 months without intervention, geriatric depression left unattended often results in complete withdrawal, confinement to bed, increased susceptibility to infection, and death. Therefore, it is essential to correctly identify geriatric depression as quickly as possible.

One of the main signs of chronic cognitive dysfunction is cognitive and intellectual impairment. Cognitive impairment includes memory deficits, disorientation to time, place, and person (in that order), loss of problem-solving skills and abstract thinking ability, impaired judgment, and a decline in intellectual ability (Angel, 1977). Unfortunately, on cursory interview, this cognitive impairment is also one of the most salient signs of severe depression as well! The severely depressed geriatric client often responds as if cognitive impairment was quite diffuse, when, in fact, there is little or no structural loss to account for this apparent impairment. The client is, presumably, too depressed to respond. When confronted with this diagnostic nightmare, the therapist has few options to follow to help differentiate.

1. The therapist should look for a precipitating event which corresponds in time to the reported onset of symptoms. This event is one which, objectively, could cause a depressive reaction. Age-related antecedents may include the loss of a spouse or sibling, loss of home, relocation, abrupt change in physical status, or forced dependency. It should be emphasized that clinicians who are not in this age group should look for *changes* of any sort, not just drastic events which they would personally perceive as possible causes of depression. A series of small changes in an elderly person's life may be sufficient, if they occur within a short time frame, to cause a depressive response. Consider the usual signs of depression such as loss of appetite, early morning awakenings, and the presence of somatic complaints (Fleiss, Gurland, & Des Roche, 1976) to aid in the differentiation.

2. Framing the questions on the mental status evaluation to purposively differentiate between depressive responding and cognitive impairment is helpful. Getting away from the standard questions regarding memory such as "Where were you born," or "Who was the President of the United States before the current one?" may help to serve this purpose. Questions from information gained from social

history or family contact which are personally relevant to the elderly client should "break through" mere poverty of response. The therapist could ask about past employment, weddings in the family, grandchildren, etc., which have more personal meaning. Keeping track of the response "I don't know," is informative since depressed individuals are more likely to respond in this manner while truly cognitively impaired individuals tend to respond more often with inappropriate or false responses. It is important to verify the information gained in this manner with other sources since recall of remote events may be disturbed.

3. The therapist should seek more sophisticated assessment devices if the picture remains cloudy. The CT scan, echoencephalogram, pneumoencephalogram, and angiogram may point out cortical losses (Wang, 1973) which may help to rule out depression alone.

4. It is important not to rely too heavily on periodic episodes of crying as a determinant of depression among elderly clients. The presence of crying is a good indicator of depression in younger age groups but crying episodes correlate highly with other conditions which are frequently present in the aged population, including cerebrovascular accidents and advanced Parkinsonism. As we have seen, crying may also be present in the chronic mental disorders as a response to periodic awareness as well.

5. If doubts still remain, it may be justifiable to ask the attending physician or psychiatrist for antidepressant medication geared toward the reduction of depression. If the cognitive impairment is reduced the problem is depression, not chronic cerebral deterioration.


## ETIOLOGY OF CHRONIC ORGANIC DISORDERS

Chronic organic dysfunction may result from a variety of causes, the end result of which appears to be cerebral cellular losses. These losses may be due to insufficient oxygen supply to brain tissue or to intrinsic destruction resulting from an unspecified virus or disease state. Commonly encountered causes include the central nervous system diseases such as Alzheimer's; abnormally progressing arteriosclerosis or atherosclerosis; infections of long duration such as syphilis and tuberculosis; nutritional deficiencies of long standing such as Vitamin $B_{12}$ or folate deficiency or general malnutrition; large subdural hematomas and resultant scarring; long-term drug and alcohol usage; anoxia secondary to heart stoppage; chronic renal, liver, or cardiac dysfunction; advanced Parkinson's disease or Huntington's chorea; uncompensated thyroid insufficiency leading to myxedema; widespread or multifocal cerebral metastasis; multifarction or thrombotic damage; and normal pressure hydrocephalus. This latter cause is thought to be modifiable, and the behavioral manifestations eliminated through the shunting of cerebrospinal fluid out from the intracranial space to other sites (Benson, 1974). The presence of ataxia and incontinence along with the usual signs of "dementia" are predictive of normal pressure hydrocephalus.

There is little difference on the behavioral level between the possible causes presented above. A few distinctions, however, have been noted and may be useful. Korsakoff's syndrome, cerebral involvement secondary to a long history of alcohol abuse, shows more striking memory impairment, confabulation, and occulargyral nystagmus than other conditions (Adams & Victor, 1970; Van Der Kolk, 1978). Impairment secondary to Alzheimer's disease typically has an earlier onset, sometimes in the middle fifties, than many of the other endogenous chronic disorders (Kent, 1977), and it and multifarct "dementia" are often slower in course than are arteriosclerotic disorders (Hachinski, Lassen, & Marshall, 1974), though this may have more to do with the age of the victims than the process alone. Hontela and Schwartz (1979) found a relationship between myocardial infarction and differing etiology. These authors noted a disproportionate number of patients with both myocardial infarctions and cerebral infarcts or hemorrhages. Patients with Alzheimer's disease show no propensity to have this cardiac problem. In the main, the behavioral results of these processes are much the same. There is significant cognitive deterioration which is often exacerbated by imposing "delirium" and the lack of social and sensory variability. These factors combine to present a clinical picture of far more impairment than one would expect with the structural damage alone. This "functional impairment" (Rossman, 1978) is the entity which needs to be properly assessed to give the complete picture of the impaired elderly client attempting to function in the environment.

## ASSESSMENT

The assessment of both acute and chronic brain disorders should involve two stages. The first stage, the behavioral level, yields signs of impaired judgment, cognitive and memory impairment, social function, reasoning ability, orientation, calculation, and arithmetic skills. These capacities are best assessed through mental status evaluations which stress functional impairment (Rossman, 1978). The Geriatric Mental Status Schedule (GMS) is specifically designed for use in the determination of the extent of impairment, whether the impairment is due to organic or functional changes, and the prediction of the course of the illness (Copeland, Kelleher, Kellett, Gourlay, Gurland, Fleiss, & Sharpe, 1976; Gurland, Copeland, Sharpe, & Kelleher, 1976). These authors have developed a structured interview format which may be administered to elderly clients in less than one hour in order to minimize fatigue. The GMS consists of between 100 and 200 questions and the rating of 500 items. Their normative studies on the GMS have yielded 21 factor scores and an inter-rater reliability value (Kappa) of .70 when used by trained psychiatrists. In addition, these authors have found that the factors of memory disorientation and cortical dysfunction load high for organically caused disorders while subjective complaints load highly for depression (Gurland et al., 1976). These authors have succeeded in making their factors mutually exclusive. Lawson, Rodenburg, and Dykes (1977) developed a dementia rating scale of 27 items which could be answered either "Yes" or "No." This scale was designed to measure orientation, emotional control, communication skills, and motor ability. The inter-rater reliability of this scale was found to be .95.

Kastenbaum and Sherwood (1972) have developed an assessment device aimed at measuring vigor, intactness, nature of relationship, and orientation based upon the interview behavior of elderly clients. Other mental status-type questionnaires designed for use with the elderly include a short-form exam developed by Pfeiffer (1975) with a test-retest correlation of .82 but some problems of intensity discrimination (Smyer, Hofland, & Jonas, 1979); a questionnaire designed specifically for assessing organic brain disorders by Fishback (1977); a Rapid Disability Rating Scale designed by Linn (1967), with an inter-rater reliability of .91 and test-retest correlation of .83; and an extended dementia scale by Hersch (1979) with a test-retest coefficient of .94. One comparison study (Haglund & Schuckit, 1976) found that the short form evaluation of Pfeiffer's correctly identified the presence of organicity more often than either a memory for designs test or a standard mental status questionnaire. But, as Kochansky (1979) suggests, further studies need to be conducted on the relative effectiveness of such tests.

While using any form of mental status examination is enlightening, the therapist should not conduct the evaluation without first acquiring a complete social history. It is impossible to accurately diagnose chronic cognitive impairment secondary to late-onset physical etiology without considering the educational history and past cognitive and intellectual level of the client. It has been this author's misfortune to feel with some confidence that a chronic, organic disorder was present in two residents of a long-term care facility. After reading the well-documented social history, however, it was found that one resident had attended school up to the second grade and the other had a long-standing diagnosis of mental retardation. It is very difficult with a one-time evaluation to see the difference between mental retardation and the results of a deterioration process in an elderly client. The length and type of prior institutionalization is also important since impaired judgment, flat or inappropriate affect, impaired cognitive processes, and a loss of self-care skills are highly correlated with long stays in mental institutions. This is an important consideration since new adaptive skills can be taught to elderly retarded individuals whereas the outcome of such training programs with progressively deteriorating clients is less optimistic. It is not enough to wait to see if the progression of the cognitive impairment makes a definitive statement regarding organic mental disorder possible, thus ruling out mental retardation. Mental retardation coupled with sensory deprivation and the sterility of many of the facilities for the elderly may lead rather rapidly to "organiclike" regression since the internal resources to counteract these negative external stimuli are not present.

One other behavioral manifestation in addition to cognitive decline is frequently encountered in chronic organic mental disorders among the elderly, particularly those which involve major cortical atrophy due to Alzheimer's disease. This behavior may best be described as "self-stimulation." In the latter stages of Alzheimer's disease, the client is often engaged in continued hand rubbing, scratching, or picking at themselves or their clothes. These clients may sit for hours in a geriatric chair rubbing table tops or rolling up their gowns, robes, or pant's legs. The following cases are descriptive of such behavior.

A seventy-one-year-old female with a diagnosis of chronic brain syndrome (DSM–II) secondary to Alzheimer's disease was referred for anxiety and agitation. She would sit up most of the day engaging in hand-washing, arm rubbing, hair pulling, and tray rubbing behavior while mumbling incoherently. Some of the tray or table-rubbing looked very much like sanding of a surface of furniture. This behavior was reduced in intensity somewhat by the administration of haloperidol 1 mg *bid.* but the behavior continues to be present. This client's EEG shows diffuse changes and slowing and the results of a CT scan show no lesions but rather the presence of diffuse atrophy.

An eighty-three-year-old female with a diagnosis of cortical atrophy exhibits a strange behavior involving taking one shoe off at a time while seated. She then rubs the inside of this shoe, puts it back on her foot, removes the other shoe, and rubs the inside of that one. This repetitive behavior may continue for hours and when interrupted by hand restraint, will continue when released.

The seventy-nine-year-old male resident of a long-term care facility presented earlier showed perseverating motor behavior which involved, first crossing one leg over the other, taking off his shoe or slipper, putting it over one hand, returning it to his foot, then crossing the other leg and repeating the motor pattern. He would also slowly and carefully roll one pantsleg up to above the knee and then back again. This behavior would continue for long periods of time when no external restraint or distractions were offered.

It may be that this type of behavior serves as sensory reinforcement for the regressed elderly individual who appears not to respond to environmental stimuli that normally produce appropriate response. Chapter 7 will include a further description of this behavior. Many such behaviors observed with these clients are similar to those self-stimulatory behaviors seen with the severely retarded and autistic children. This parallel needs exploration.

The second level of assessment is physical evaluation. Some of these somatic techniques have been mentioned before in connection with differential diagnosis and include the electroencephalogram, echoencephalogram, computerized axial tomography, and the angiogram (Wang, 1973). Physical diagnosis is often costly, painful, and intrusive. The main drawback may be that the therapist will be deterred from instituting active therapy if significant anatomical pathology is found. However, it is the most fundamental assessment approach in that it may provide definitive proof of underlying cerebral or vascular damage. Neurological consultation often proves to be valuable as well. Focal tissue dysfunction due to trauma, infarct, or neoplasms, may present initially as more diffuse, and amorphous decline when combined with the client's maladaptive behavior in response to the changes brought about by this focal damage. Withdrawal, depression, and excess disability may confuse the clinical picture to such an extent that the therapist may assume that global and diffuse brain involvement is present. The presence of communication disorders secondary to cerebral damage, particularly global aphasia, may offer another source of confusion in assessment. Aphasia, which may result in sing-song, repetitive, nonsensical speech, could easily be confused with schizophrenic jargon complete with neologisms. Consultation with a speech pathologist or neurologist could prevent a gross error in diagnosis. Visual or auditory deficits, previously undetected, may confound the presentation of symptoms. The presence of these sensory deficits may be complicated by denial of sensory decrements on the part of the elderly client or the lack of familiarity with common prosthetic devices such as cataract glasses and hearing aides. One client, with whom the author is familiar, was referred by nursing personnel of a long-term care facility for progressively more frequent delusions and hallucinations. The clinical psychologist referred this client to the speech pathologist for a hearing screening and the results of this testing led to a referral to the physician. The client, whose hygiene behavior was far from adequate, was found to have an enormous wax buildup in his ears. When this was evacuated, the client exhibited no further signs of inappropriate behavior.

Working with the elderly, one begins to marvel at the complexity of the assessment issue. There is no other client population this size which presents more diverse causative possibilities, including those endogenous antecedents of which most psychologists are less than familiar. The psychologist interested in working with the geriatric client must have an extensive acquaintance with a variety of scientific areas including sensory psychology, perception, physiology, speech pathology, pharmacology, medicine, neuroanatomy, and nutrition.

If clinical assessment is detective work, then assessment with elderly clients is the ultimate whodunit. The challenge of this unraveling process comes from the complexity of variables including the high incidence of behavioral and organic process interactions, idiosyncratic drug responses, nonuniform sensory decrements across individuals and modalities, the increased variability in behavioral responses due to longer conditioning histories, differences in the environments in which the elderly often find themselves, and the vast number of changes of all types which the elderly must face. If the negative connotations which surround the aging process and correlated illnesses are somehow removed or reduced, the influx of psychologists into geriatrics should be immense just for the excitement and challenge this population has to offer. It is hoped that the remainder of this book will help to reduce these negative connotations, for even a minor show of interest would be welcomed.

# 5
# Assessment: An Analysis of Functional Variables

Functional analysis provides the clinical assessor with a valuable guide in the case-by-case analysis of nonorganic relationships with the elderly. It also provides a convenient summary device for the more general description of frequently encountered problems in the elderly group as a whole. An example of functional analysis is shown as Figure 5-1. This figure gives the reader a framework to more easily proceed through this chapter and should be referred to as needed. As will become clear, such a delineation is somewhat arbitrary and many of the factors involved in the assessment of geriatric clients may be seen to fit several categories. For example, accelerated tissue atrophy in the brain has been shown to be so reliably correlated with abnormal behavioral manifestations as to be considered a "stimulus" variable. Since this tissue pathology is within the individual it may also be considered an "organism" variable as well.

However, some researchers argue that tissue atrophy may well be caused by another commonly occurring "stimulus" variable, sensory deprivation or isolation, thereby making such damage a "response" variable. To complicate the picture further, tissue loss may also be seen as a "consequence" of withdrawal, withdrawal being the response to perceived helplessness and a cause of sensory deprivation. Hence, tissue loss is a "consequence" variable as well.

| Stimuli | Organism Variables | Responses | Consequences |
|---------|--------------------|-----------|--------------| 
| Isolation | *Physiological* | Withdrawal | Institutionalization |
| Sensory deprivation | Tissue atrophy | Depression | Further decline |
| Social losses | Central slowing | Suspiciousness | Tissue atrophy |
| Society's attitudes | *Cognitive* | Complaints | Avoidance by others |
|  | Worthlessness | Attention-seeking |  |
|  | Passive acceptance | Skills suppression |  |
|  | "I won't try that | "Chronic brain |  |
|  | again!" | syndrome" |  |
|  | Loss of control |  |  |
|  | "Learned helplessness" |  |  |

Note: As discussed in the text, most of these subvariables may fall into more than one category and may be both a cause and a result of other subvariables.

Figure 5-1.    Functional Analysis of Geriatric Behavior.

## CHRONIC NONORGANIC CHANGES

Organic etiologies of behavioral abnormalities are present more frequently in the geriatric population than in other age groups. It does not necessarily follow though that organicity is the most frequent cause of behavioral abnormalities in the geriatric population. The main diagnostic problem lies in the fact that many of the observed behavioral problems among the elderly involve *interactions* between organic (physical) and nonorganic (functional) factors.

Unfortunately, the DSM-I and DSM-II classification systems, in an attempt to deal with this complicated assessment picture, have provided the clinician with a label of dubious, if not iatrogenic, value: Chronic brain syndrome. This nomenclature is supposed to describe the symptom complex which includes a general decline in cognitive functioning, disorientation, confusion, multiple memory dysfunctions, decrease in inhibitory control, and a general deterioration of hygiene concerns. The label is applied when all of the following criteria are present.

1.   Advanced chronological age.
2.   General gradual decline in the appropriateness of the functions described above with no definite precipitating factor (e.g., long-term alcohol abuse).

3.  No hard evidence of organic etiology is present. This includes an absence of tumors, cerebral infarcts, chronic diseases, hematomas, cortical lesions, or distinct cortical atrophy.

The assignment of this label has perhaps been the most grievous error in the assessment and treatment of adult psychopathology. Not only does the label "chronic brain syndrome" suggest nothing of etiology or specific treatment, but its application has usually meant the premature termination of the assessment-treatment process. Since the description of the commonly presenting symptoms are similar to those described in Chapter 4 which result from treatable causes, the tragedy is readily apparent. The fact that custodial placement often follows the display of such behavior and such placement often effectively eliminates exposure to appropriate treatment methods, adds to the poignancy of the elderly person's predicament. In fact, it is the nature of such "treatment" which has recently been implicated as a causal variable in the maintenance of chronic nonorganic and organic dysfunction. Isolation and sensory-stimuli reduction are two of the main precipitating factors.

## Stimuli Reduction and Chronic Change

Ernst and his colleagues (Ernst, Badash, Beran, Kosovsky, & Kleinhauz, 1977; Ernst, Beran, Badash, Kosovsky, & Kleinhauz, 1977; Ernst, Beran, & Kleinhauz, 1979; Ernst, Beran, Safford, & Kleinhauz, 1978) have suggested that the behavioral manifestations which are often labeled as chronic brain syndrome may or may not involve tissue pathology. Regardless, the more appropriate target for change is isolation. Isolation is not only more easily modifiable, but also may occur earlier in the chain of causation than tissue pathology. It is also possible that isolation is the important factor in determining whether or not a given amount of tissue loss will result in noticeable alterations in behavior.

What we *are* suggesting is the following: since CBS is a multifactorial disease and since we do not precisely know the degree of brain damage present, nor can we at the present time do very much about whatever brain deterioration is present, it is best to work with the isolation factor. (Ernst, Beran, & Kleinhauz, 1979, pp. 531–532)

In terms of assessment, therefore, it is imperative to entertain the complex interrelationship between organicity and those functional variables which are often present in the elderly person's environment. Arguments involving the relative importance of functional versus organic etiologies in the development of chronic behavior problems only detract from the significant applied task of complete assessment and treatment and would probably result in an outcome resembling the tiring nature-nurture controversy. It should be sufficient to concern oneself with the fact that, whether or not tissue pathology is present, isolation and sensory deprivation may result in those behavioral manifestations which as a group have been labeled as chronic brain syndrome.

Research has indicated that visual deprivation leads to changes in the visual cortex, olfactory deprivation reduces olfactory bulb growth, and tactile stimulation-reduction leads to changes in blood-plasma levels of various hormonal substances in animals. Dendritic branching and axonal growth have long been known to be retarded by severe isolation from sensory stimuli. With impaired structure it is reasonable to assume that behavior and perceptual processes will also be detrimentally effected.

Behavioral assessment, then, should include an analysis of the context in which the disordered behavior occurs. Such an analysis should include the following.

1. Any recent reductions in the number or quality of social contacts prior to the behavior change. A reduction in or total elimination of social contacts results in the absence of feedback from others regarding the appropriateness of one's behavior. Social relations also contain an informational component which, when unavailable couple with a reduction in the auditory and visual capabilities, resulting in a decrease in the total amount of information necessary to conduct one's day-to-day affairs. Minor difficulties may gradually compound to result in inadequate response if a significant other is not present to intervene or to prompt the elderly person to utilize appropriate coping strategies.

2. A recent relocation to a new residence regardless of the number

of new contacts of a social nature. Oftentimes an elderly individual does not benefit from potential new social contacts because previously unneeded social skills have not developed. Also, because of fears of ambulating in architecturally different physical settings and the unfamiliarity of routine activities, the client may feel less comfortable in interacting with social contacts or the new environment even though much care went into the design of such environments.

3. The results of physical examinations which reveal developing cataracts, worsening visual acuity, worsening auditory acuity, or increasing mobility limitations. These conditions suggest that the client is not only receiving less environmental information and stimulation, but may also be reacting to these new limitations in a self-defeating manner. Various adaptive devices may have been prescribed for these limitations but some elderly individuals fail to achieve the maximum utility of these items either because of discomfort, poor technical information, denial of the need for such instrumentation, or forgetfulness.

4. The location of residence and the quality of the stimulation must also be considered. Poverty or medical necessity may have resulted in less than adequate surroundings which are minimally stimulating or reinforcing. Careful consideration to the stimulus elements of the client's residence should include the level of functioning of other residents in the vicinity, access to and utilization of activities, media sources, ongoing visual and auditory cues, and ease of ambulation.

5. The possibility of depression or other affective disorders must be considered. Just as chronic changes secondary to organic involvement often present much the same as depression or anxiety so, too, do nonorganic changes. Some of the same guidelines in differential diagnosis described in Chapter 4 should be helpful in this regard. Depression *as a cause of chronic deterioration* should also be considered since depression in the elderly often leads to social isolation and withdrawal from ongoing activities.

## Loss of Control and Responsibility

Chronic change complete with disorientation, memory loss, physical losses, and inattention to personal appearance may also result from response to external control. This subjective loss of control over the antecedents and consequences of one's own behavior which, in time, results in withdrawal and inappropriate response is similar to Seligman's concept of "learned helplessness." This term describes an acquired pattern of response to stressful situations after previous experience in similar situations. In the earlier situation the ability to escape stress was prevented. The fact that one's behavior in the situation where the stress was inescapable had no effect on changing the situation is thought to be an analogue of helplessness. The resulting response takes the form of passivity, withdrawal, anxiety, and totally inadequate behavior. It is not difficult to equate the situation in which many elderly individuals find themselves (i.e., nursing homes, hospitals, relatives' homes) with the experimentally induced situation where one's behavior has little or no effect on the situation and the locus of all control is external.

A recent study by Rodin and Langer (1977) showed that elderly residents of a nursing home who were initially matched according to physical health and other variables, differed on post-test measures of confusion and well-being consequent to different levels of self-control. The seemingly trivial task of caring for indoor plants was either left to the residents or was undertaken by the staff. The subjects who had to take care of the plants showed less confusion and less psychological difficulties, and even a lower mortality rate on an eighteen-month follow-up, than those who were given the plants but not the task of caring for them. Therefore, in this one rather small area of control or responsibility, significant differences appeared on behavioral measures.

Langer, Rodin, Beck, Weinman, and Spitzer (1978) showed that both short-term and long-term memory was more positively affected by a nursing home environment in which the residents were required to attend to their needs (more demanding) than those who had their needs constantly attended to by others (less demanding). It is thought that manipulations of the demanding nature of the residential environment is one aspect of manipulating locus of control. By "allowing" the elderly resident to control the contingencies over their own behavior, the usual manifestations of chronic brain syndrome appear to lessen.

It has recently been argued that the symptoms commonly referred to as chronic brain syndrome are not natural consequences to aging. This enlightened approach emphasizes that this symptom complex is neither statistically frequent nor an automatic correlate. Although this attitude is a welcome change in that it leads to more active intervention and more optimism regarding the entire aging process, it is in a way misleading. Growing old *does* often result in the aforementioned behavior and given the factors of social isolation, sensory deprivation, endogenous correlative changes, and loss of control, much of the inappropriate behavior observed in this population is a *natural* occurrence. If we define natural as understandable or reliably occurring and if the process is left to occur without some type of intervention, abnormal behavior *should* occur. Rather than removing all considerations of such negative adaptations we should incorporate them continually in our formulation of geriatric psychopathology. When we view the frequently encountered problems of the elderly as understandable responses to naturally occurring externally induced changes we may be able to understand the functional relationships between, not only chronic brain syndrome and the aging process, but also other high frequency problematic behavior such as depression, paranoia, hypochondriasis, anxiety, and skills deficits. When these responses are present appropriate compensatory behavior may be prevented.

## DEPRESSION IN THE GERIATRIC POPULATION

Depression is the number one psychopathological condition among the elderly and is by far the most widely encountered set of abnormal behaviors encountered in facilities for the aged. Depression presents less clear-cut symptomatology (Epstein, 1978) in the elderly age group than in younger populations. Geriatric depression often appears to present shallower symptoms with more chronicity than found in younger people (Goldstein, 1979). Typically, the depressed elderly client shows more biological involvement including insomnia, anorexia, weight loss, and "depressive equivalents." This latter concept describes the emergence of depression in the form of multiple somatic complaints often involving the gastrointestinal system and urinary tract disorders (Salzman & Shader, 1978). As a matter of fact, hypochondriasis, which is also encountered frequently with the aged population, is thought to result at least partially from an underlying depression. Hypochondriacal response is but one form of attention-seeking aimed at the reduction of depression through increasing social contact and social reinforcement.

In addition to the relatively frequent physical involvement, depression in the elderly also presents the same symptoms as depression in any age group, such as sadness, withdrawal, pessimism, apathy, and, sometimes, agitation (Pfeiffer & Busse, 1969). As Epstein (1976, p. 278) states:

> *The implication of recognizing that such manifestations are symptoms of depressive illness in the elderly lies in the fact that with appropriate treatment, depressive symptoms generally have a favorable prognosis.*

Not only is the outcome of appropriately diagnosed depression favorable, but mistakes in the assessment process which results in not targeting depression may well lead to further decline. Unlike depression occurring in younger populations, geriatric depression does not remit as frequently without intervention and may result in a slowing of bodily functions to the point of death.

The main correlative behavior of depression in the elderly, which distinguishes it from depression in younger clients, is the apparent confusion or cloudiness of cognitive functioning. Along with the common dulling of affect is a dulling of intellectual functioning, less attention to personal hygiene and appearance, and moderate levels of disorientation. It may be remembered from Chapter 4 that it is this cognitive and intellectual involvement which contributes to the confusion in the differential diagnosis of geriatric depression and cerebral losses. Special care must be taken to analyze any functional variables such as drastic losses in reinforcement, decreases in the activity level, relocation, loss of a significant other, or increasing physical limitations so that the label of chronic deterioration is not automatically invoked. Persistent questioning should help to determine if unresponsiveness to items on mental status exams and tests of intellectual function is due to true deficits or lack of motivation to respond.

Many functional causes of depression have been offered. Freud viewed depression as due to a "loss of an ambivalently held introjected love object" and Levin offers a "libido in search of gratification" (Peak, 1972, p. 167). In the elderly, Lipton (1976) has suggested that increased monoamineoxidase activity leads to a decrease in amines at the synapses which, in turn, leads to depression. Genetic theories (Mendlewicz, 1976) which stress the importance of predisposition suggest that taking an accurate family history during assessment is beneficial. However, in keeping with our compensatory model, other hypotheses are suggested to explain the high frequency of depressive behavior in the elderly population. These include the following:

1. The normal correlative changes in the aging process may lead to depressive responding if the individual is not properly prepared and misattributes these decreases in the quality of function for atypical deterioration. Questions which involve the individual's perception of aging or a description by that individual of elderly acquaintances may help to uncover such causative misperceptions.

2. Accelerated cerebral tissue loss which is perceived by the elderly individual may lead to responses which appear as depressive reactions. Instead of positively coping with behavioral and cognitive deficits an understandable, though less constructive response, might be to avoid daily activities and routines, thus underemphasizing the decreased function. This avoidance results in situations in which these deficits in response do not meet with adverse consequences. Such reductions in social contacts and activity level rapidly become self-fulfilling.

The assessor may pinpoint this functional cause by assessing the earlier coping strategies of the elderly client. If there is a history of less than adequate response to change or stress the interviewer should suspect inadequate coping ability (Fassler & Gaviria, 1978). Past inadequacies will be exaggerated with aging since the ability to compensate for change decreases even more with advancing years.

3. Increased reliance on others, due to personal limitations or residence-induced removal of control, may lead to feelings of hopelessness, loss of control, further dependency on others for the basics of life, and a type of "learned helplessness." When others are providing everything including decision-making, there is no reason to actively engage in those activities which are incompatible with depression. Flat affect and apathy are natural consequences of such behavior. The interviewer should include questions regarding locus of

control and the relative importance assigned to others in the life of the elderly client. Questions such as, "Who decides if and when you go shopping?", and "Why do you go to bed when you do?", may help to fix perceived locus of control.

Several standardized assessment devices designed to measure depression are available. The Geriatric Mental Status interview (Kelleher, Copeland, Gurland, & Sharpe, 1976) and the Philadelphia Geriatric Center Morale Scale (Lawton, 1972) are two possible candidates. The latter includes 41 items with test-retest correlations of between .75 and .91 and internal consistency of .81. The best scale may well be the Beck Depression Inventory (Beck, Ward, Mendelson, Mock, & Erbaugh, 1961) even though it was not specifically designed for use with geriatric populations. This scale contains 21 items in a multiple-choice format.

The Beck Inventory is particularly sensitive in measuring geriatric depression because it contains many items with somatic references such as amount of sleep, feelings of fatigue, appetite, weight loss, concerns regarding personal health, personal attractiveness, and interest in sex. Although it is not advocated that one attach an overall score to any individual (thus suggesting some trait or depressive personality type) an individual item-analysis of the responses may prove useful in the assessment of the intensity of depressive response and any changes attributable to treatment. Responses on the Beck Inventory, coupled with naturalistic observations, interview data, and ratings by family or staff members may combine to give an accurate picture of the parameters of the depression.

## Activity Level and Depression

Activity level is a particularly good indicator of depression among the elderly and one that is subject to quantification. Gross measures such as the number of activities attended (with reference to a baseline measure) may be easily documented by activities personnel or family members. In more extreme cases, the number of hours in bed during the day, time spent in the client's bedroom, or the number of feet traveled during an eight-hour shift are useful predictors of depressive reactions. Being discrete and countable, these are ideal measures for assessing the efficacy of treatment programs as well. Though they tend to require more diligence on the part of the observers, they reflect withdrawal and inactivity with sensitivity.

A seventy-two-year old man with diagnoses of schizophrenia, chronic undifferentiated type, and diabetes mellitus periodically complained of being tired, stomach upset, and sadness while residing in a nursing home. Concomitantly, he would quit participating in special activities and social contacts which were normally maintained at a high rate.

An observer recorded on floor plans the number of feet covered in one hour outside of his room at random times during the day. Spot-check reliability was taken by another trained observer. After one week of baseline data was compiled, a gradual shaping procedure was introduced using the number of feet traveled as the dependent measure of treatment success. Once the shaping program had affected his behavior such that he had returned to one activity, the distance measure was terminated and the number of activities became the target of the shaping procedure. One beneficial side-effect of having staff act as observers has been that the client's early withdrawal behavior has come to elicit concern in the staff members and the shaping procedure is quickly reactivated before the more regressed response (remaining in room) is exhibited.

Behavioral theoreticians involved with depression usually concentrate on the lack of activity inherent in depressive responding. Lewinsohn and Graf (1973), for example, emphasize the need for reinforcement programs to increase activity level which, in turn, alleviate depression. Though it cannot be argued that activity level does appear to be correlated with levels of depression, it is but one aspect of such behavior and should not be the sole assessment measure nor the sole criterion for treatment efficacy. To argue that depression is often accompanied by lowered activity levels and that correction of this one component is equivalent to a reduction in depression is an oversimplification. Other measures of depression must be attended to in the assessment-treatment process. These other measures include observer-rated affect, self-reported depression, changes in the biological functioning (sleeping, eating, and sexual patterns of behavior), the content of speech, and cognitive behavior. This latter component requires additional attention.

## Cognitive Correlates and Depression

Another array of behaviors which, when properly considered, helps signal the presence or absence of depression, is the cognitive component. This is not to argue that this source of depressive equivalence is relatively more important in the development or assessment of depression than other correlates, but that thought patterns may be indicative of depression even when more readily observable correlates are not evident. In the geriatric client, expressions of loneliness, worthlessness, and sadness often occur *before* the more obvious behaviors of avoidance and reduced participation in ongoing activities. Such verbalizations may represent stimuli meant to elicit attention or special favors from significant others, but their association with geriatric depression is too strong to be overlooked.

The assessor should be particularly alert to statements incorporating references to no longer being in control of things or being under the control of others. These statements suggest that the directionality of all activities, rewards, feedback, and control is one-sided. These statements are often the initial signs in a chain which terminates in complete passive acceptance and a low level of responsivity. Maladaptive cognitive behaviors are targets for change in their own right, as well.

The amount of self-talk among the elderly is striking. Often these covert statements become verbalized in the course of daily routine and the frequency of negative, self-defeating statements is unnerving. While performing simple tasks in the presence of an observer many irrational overgeneralizations are made usually in reference to loss of ability and decreased adequacy. Unfortunately, these statements often interfere with the performance of the task by distracting the elderly client from pertinent cues. When the task is not completed or is completed poorly, these negative self-evaluations are reinforced. During assessment it is important to gain access to this maladaptive dialogue in an attempt to gain a complete picture of the inappropriate behavior. However, depression is but one problematic behavior in which negative self-statements are abundant.

## PARANOID BEHAVIOR

Another high-frequency behavior found in the elderly population is paranoid thought. This suspiciousness is neither an age-related trait nor a natural tendency of an age-group which has gotten out-of-hand. However, this behavior is understandable and predictable given the compensatory model and functional analysis. Consider an elderly individual who is experiencing some difficulty in visual and auditory acuity who is uprooted from his/her place of long-term residence for a room in a geriatric facility or is repeatedly moved from one relative's home to another. Added to this are the complicating factors of distasteful medicine, strange food cooked by others, slight disorientation, and forgetfulness regarding the location of common objects such as glasses, canes, and wearing apparel. If familiar and trustworthy social contacts are no longer present, correcting feedback is limited. The aches and pains of bodily systems which accompanies normal aging become intensified because activities and stimulation may be limited. A typical response to a combination of these factors is suspiciousness.

Paranoid ideation in the elderly is slightly different from that of full-blown paranoia in younger cohorts in that the targets of the delusional thinking are usually persons in the immediate environment and in close contact with the client rather than extraterrestials or electronic devices (Pfeiffer & Busse, 1969). All in all, the understandable, albeit inappropriate responses, are a range of feelings including "those around me no longer care," and feelings of active persecution. Suspiciousness, then, takes on an adaptive function for these clients. The behavior essentially is a protective device, a defense against actual "harm." A sampling of actual thoughts is illustrative.

1. "My children put me here to get me out of the way. They just wanted my lovely home."
2. "This food here is making me sick. They put a purgative in the food, gives me diarrhea."
3. "The nurses don't like me. They never answer my light. They try to poison me with that green medicine, but I won't take it."
4. "I heard them say that they're going to kill me tonight. A man came into my room last night and told me they wanted me dead."

These thoughts appear to be entirely irrational but usually the basis for the illogical thinking is partially true. Very seldom will an entirely unrealistic statement be made that, with some diligence, cannot be discovered to have originated or been maintained by true occurrences. Nursing personnel monitoring physical signs during the night become assassins. Barely audible voices or fragments of loudspeaker announcements become personalized. Roommates whisked away during the night are victims of a private curse which, for the present, somehow missed the appropriate target. Unfortunately, a common response of others on continually hearing such talk is avoidance, thus eliminating more completely any access to realistic feedback and reality testing. Even more pills or larger pills are soon provided, the client's name is mentioned more often by persons passing by, and restraints for the client's safety may be prescribed in order to prevent possibilities of injury due to mental deterioration. The delusion, which started as a result of impaired acuity or unwanted relocation, soon becomes elaborately and frighteningly ubiquitous. One case should serve as an example.

A seventy-seven-year old female patient had recently been admitted to an intermediate-care facility from her home. When interviewed by a variety of staff members she recounted a bizarre and incredible story of being held prisoner in her own home for weeks by a group of young people. These captors supposedly kept her in a closet, bound, and barely nourished while they ransacked her house, intercepted her mail and entertained friends. No amount of persuasion or rational argument could dissuade the patient's story though careful checking proved the story completely false. What was almost accidentally discovered however was that the patient had been resuscitated by an emergency rescue team following cardiac arrest and syncope which had led to the nursing home placement. She had had the attack while watching a television program about the Manson family crimes. It is thought that, in the confusion during the episode, she had assimilated bits and pieces of the program to her own situation.

It is also often the case that some of the high incidence of paranoid behavior attributed to the elderly may be, in part, due to the misperceptions of the observers. More than one case of suspected paranoia has been determined at some point to be quite realistic. The "crazy lady" down the block who swears that people are taunting her while hiding in her shrubs at night or the rest home resident who is sure that someone is spying on her when she undresses at night have sometimes been vindicated. The neighborhood kids out to see a real eccentric or the man down the hall whose approach to sexual release is limited have been discovered to be real entities. Unfortunately, action may have been taken to "protect" the elderly client before such factors have come to light.

Several considerations should be incorporated in the assessment of such problematic behavior. As might be imagined, separation of paranoid behavior and attention-seeking is a difficult process given the hesitancy of such individuals to share their experiences. Such differentiation is extremely important, however, since the choice of treatment and probability of success is quite different.

1. Unless the paranoid thought is ridiculously bizarre, it is probably best to regard such reports as being, at least in part, true. If the client persists in the face of contrary evidence to stick to the misperception, action may be taken. Care must be taken to account for all possible objective causes of such thoughts. Do the people in the next room fight, curse, threaten, or laugh out loud a lot? Could an insensitive staff or family member threaten incarceration or restraint or worse out of frustration or hostility? Are there several such patients on the same hall or do they spend time socializing a lot? Had there been a particularly graphic television program containing subject matter closely related to the "delusion" which coincides with the first report of the "delusion?" Has the client recently been exposed to a particularly persuasive religious presentation either in the media or in local churches? Any of these questions may help to highlight potential causes of paranoid thought.

2. Some verbalizations may represent attention-seeking behavior on the part of the elderly client. Complaints that no one cares anymore or someone is out to get them usually result, at least initially, in a positive response on the part of others. The responses of others, then, serve to maintain the verbal behavior on the part of the client. It is necessary to differentiate between this attempt for attention and suspiciousness and irrational thinking. In-depth probing of the "delu-

sional" content should help discern the difference. It is also more likely that a truly suspicious person will not easily verbalize to the mental health professional details of a conspiracy until he or she is quite sure that the professional is not in on the plot. Information too readily given and conversation which is volunteered by the client should lead one to conclude that the behavior is elicited to gain attention.

## HYPOCHONDRIACAL BEHAVIOR

The verbal expression of multiple somatic complaints with no organic etiology is quite common among the elderly. It is so common that chronic complaining has become a part of the stereotyped picture of an old person. Again, this is a set of behaviors which may be seen in light of the compensatory model. The elderly individual *does* experience a variety of physical ailments during the senescent period. These aches, pains, and changes, when accompanied by verbal expression often result in prompt attention, soothing words, and contact with individuals not normally seen on a routine basis (i.e., physicians, licensed nursing personnel, out-of-town family members, mental health practitioners, or a usually disinterested relative). Unfortunately, due to the death of friends and the ignorance of younger persons, positive social consequences may result *only when such verbalizations are made.* More positive attempts to receive social reinforcement or attention may have failed.

Hypochondriacal behavior may also result from preoccupation with bodily concerns. This can easily result in geriatric facilities with a medical atmosphere. The "ravages of aging" are known to the client. Friends and acquaintances in the facility are continually sick or they are dying, the usual forms of distraction and coping are not available, and the client may well be experiencing discomfort from a variety of causes, real or imagined. Against the backdrop of little stimulation one's bodily changes become exaggerated.

Other theories, somewhat related to the idea of inappropriate compensation to natural occurrences have been developed. Walsh (1976), for example, views hypochondriasis as a result of a chain of situations. The elderly person has impaired circulation in the brain due to the concomitants of aging or accelerated circulatory loss. This impedance in circulation is thought to lower adaptation to problem situations when they occur, leading to stress and anxiety. This anxiety takes the form of concentration on minor bodily changes which are verbalized to such an extent that very little else is thought about or said. This fits in with our overall notion of impaired adaptability and the inappropriate behavior which may result from inflexibility.

Brink (1978) and Brink, Capri, DeNeeve, Janakes, and Oliveira (1979) view hypochondriasis as a defense mechanism of the elderly. They cite their finding that hypochondriasis and paranoid ideation frequently occur together, the correlation being +.45. In confused clients, heightened suspiciousness and overconcern about the body are natural responses to poor adjustment, the rigors of growing old and loss of control. In order to regain some control over their surroundings, paranoid thoughts and somatic complaints serve to gain the attention of others. This would lead to a situation of natural reinforcement of the inappropriate behavior. Their findings and resultant theorizing also fit nicely with the compensatory model. These two sets of behaviors are ways to regain control which has been lost or taken away due to the lowered status of the elderly client.

Support for this idea is provided by Busse (1976) who found that hypochondriasis is correlated with lower socioeconomic status, increased levels of stress, dependency, loss of role status, poor physical health, and marital discord. Busse suggests that hypochondriacal behavior is a form of improper compensation to these aversive situations.

Therefore, it is plausible to view the verbalization of multiple somatic complaints as a compensatory behavior. The elderly individual who expresses these complaints, then, is attempting to regain some control over the situations and persons around them and to behave in such a way increases the likelihood of receiving stimulation and positive reinforcement from the environment. The fact that such behavior is judged to be inappropriate does not detract from the fact that it is predictable in the situations that many elderly persons find themselves.

A scale for use in the assessment of hypochondriasis has recently been developed by Brink, Belanger, Bryant, Capri, Janakes, Jasculca, and Oliveira (1978). This scale, the Hypochondriasis Scale for Institutionalized Geriatrics, was tested on a sample of 10 subjects who were diagnosed as hypochondriacal and 59 control subjects in an extended-care facility. The raters were blind to the diagnoses. Questions on this scale include, "Do you feel your best in the morning?", "Are you satisfied with your health most of the time?", and "Is it hard for you to believe it when the nurse tells you that there is nothing physically wrong with you?"

The score on this in-patient scale revealed significant differences in response between the hypochondriacal subjects and the nonhypochondriacal controls. The only drawback of the use of this scale is that it yields many false positive results, so it should be used with care and only in conjunction with interview, observational, and other data.

Some considerations in the assessment of possible hypochondriacal behavior include the following:

1. One should, at least initially, assume that the physical complaint does, indeed, have a basis in organicity. This would be the case unless reliable medical testimony is to the contrary or the complaints have occurred over a time-span of years. The presence of physical changes, as has been mentioned, is omnipresent and some of the manifestations of such changes in the elderly are quite different from those in other age groups. Unwanted medication side-effects, poorly fixated descriptions of discomfort, and poor memory for onset may complicate the picture.

The services of a physician should be sought. It should be noted, too, that the discovery of a medical problem does not mean that the search for other physical etiologies should stop, nor that the complaints will quickly be resolved if the source of physical discomfort is alleviated. In our analysis of one possible way in which hypochondriacal behavior could be maintained we discussed the role of the attention paid by others consequent to the verbalization of somatic complaints. It may be that the real physical problem has provided a means to attract this attention so the probability that such a strategy will be utilized by the elderly client again is high. In other words, if it worked before, it should continue to work. This is of course a behavioral view of "secondary gain."

2. The assessor should observe the responses of others to the verbalization of the somatic complaints and also their behavior toward

the client when he or she is not making such complaints. If the difference is striking, one might suspect that the behavior of others is maintaining the chronic complaints. Again, this does not rule out the possibility of organic involvement.

3. A valuable tool in the assessment of possible hypochondriacal behavior involves the dual role of assessment and treatment. By providing other outlets for the client for attention-seeking and by reinforcing more appropriate behavior, one should see a decline in the number of complaints if organicity does not exist. If there exists a real physical cause for the behavior the complaints should not decrease substantially.

4. A long history of chronic complaints, and the presence of complaints involving nonsomatic topics is helpful in differentiating between hypochondriasis and justifiable complaints. There is a high probability that the chronic complainer will also verbalize his or her displeasure with the conduct of other persons around them, the quality of nursing care, the involvement of family and friends, the quality of the food, the temperature, the lighting, and any number of environmental components. If such varied complaints are also present, one should suspect inappropriate attention-seeking and not a medical cause.

5. One should note the onset of the somatic complaints as well. Though such verbalizations may be modeled and may present with some suddenness if others are receiving attention by expressing certain symptoms, hypochondriasis usually does not appear overnight. Also, if the complaint occurs reliably at certain times of the day or after certain activities, the discreteness of the onset may indicate physical involvement. If the complaint is voiced only in the morning, after meals, after or before urination or elimination, after climbing stairs, after physical therapy, or at night, a physical cause should be suspected. However, hypochondriasis may also be viewed as an avoidance behavior, as a way of getting out of doing things which are bothersome or tiring. Anyone who has witnessed an elderly client prior to his/her appointment in physical therapy is well aware of the increase in physical ailments at that time. Therefore, it is important to consider the possibility of the relative reinforcement derived from avoidance.

## ANXIETY

Another response-competitor which should be assessed when skills appear deficient is anxiety. Anxiety in geriatric clients, which is thought to occur with great frequency (Oberleder, 1966), differs little from anxiety manifested by younger clients. However, anxiety due to misattribution is almost solely a geriatric response. Also, there are some stimulus elements which are more often anxiety-producing in the elderly population than in younger samples.

Oftentimes, elderly clients will complain of being anxious or nervous by indicating obvious limb tremors, restlessness, inability to sleep, or an inability to concentrate. The content of thought is something like, "I am nervous because I am shaking, restless, etc." These complaints are seen as symptoms of an underlying nervous state or condition. The assessors first task, though, is to determine the proper sequence of events. Often, it is not some state of nervousness or anxiety which is resulting in these aforementioned symptoms, but rather the exhibition of these behavioral manifestations which is *causing* anxiety. The true source of these symptoms may be a medication or physical disorder such as Parkinsonism which is being mislabeled by the elderly client as anxiety. In fact, anxiety may well be present as a result of recognizing the manifestations and becoming concerned about them.

The interviewer should consult the client's drug regimen and medical diagnoses to rule out a physiological basis for the symptoms.

Of course, the reported or observed anxiety may well be a result of nonorganic stimuli just as with younger persons. These age-related anxiety-producing stimuli not only include the common objects and situations which plague other age groups, such as insects, the sight of blood, strangers, and elevators, but may also include changes in residence, fears of losing control, financial problems, death and dying, being alone, stairways, steps, going outdoors alone, being too far away from a bathroom, inability to remember recent or remote events with any clarity, spending holidays alone, fear of postholiday depression, losing one's sensory acuity, losing one's mind, choking, being robbed or accosted, being laughed at, various modes of transportation, going shopping, physical examinations, and minor surgery. All of these situations may pose serious threats to an elderly, slightly incapacitated person for very good reasons. As a matter of fact, the bizarre, totally irrational fears often encountered in clinical practice with younger clientele are seldom found with the elderly. It may be that totally irrational fears have been selected out by mortality or have been supplanted by more ubiquitous, yet understandable fears. It just doesn't seem that there are any elderly snake phobics seeking contact with therapists.

It is also more difficult to find discrete, limited stimuli as causes of anxiety with this age group. Pervasive anxiety is more frequent in the geriatric population. Either because of numerous fear-provoking stimuli in their environment, internal changes causing nebulous anxiety, or one or two ever-present and inescapable fear-provoking stimuli (e.g., physical incapacitation, loss of control, death) it is more difficult finding the easily delineated phobic object or situation. The therapist should be attending to this global, perfuse anxiety in the assessment. When presented with an elderly client who has difficulty in narrowing down the times, places, or events in which he or she experiences anxiety and when responses to questions are similar to those of a depressed client, one should consider this nondiscrete anxiety. Restlessness and akathisia during the interview help to differentiate chronic anxiety (or drug effect) from depression.

Anxiety, hypochondriasis, suspiciousness (paranoid behavior) and depression are commonly encountered problems with elderly clients. These behaviors compete with behavior which is more constructive, goal-directed, and adaptive. Accurate assessment is necessary in order, not only to differentiate these competing responses from chronic organic deterioration, but also from response inadequacy due to inefficient compensatory skills.

## SKILLS LOSS AND SKILLS SUPPRESSION

An individual's ability to interact with the environment is based, in large part, on his or her competency. Competency is most usefully defined as the presence of skills requisite for adequate daily functioning as well as the adaptability to successfully deal with new stimulus situations without inappropriate responses of anxiety or depression. In the geriatric population less than competent responding to problematic situations or daily activities results in behavioral manifestations such as poor hygiene, withdrawal, anxiety, depression, suspiciousness, inappropriate attention-seeking behavior, and inappropriate social and sexual behavior.

Poor adaptive skills may result from either of four causes. First, the elderly individual may never have learned competent adaptive skills or may possess only marginally effective skills and therefore would not exhibit those skills currently. Second, other responses such as anxiety, physical limitations, or depression may have suppressed skills that the elderly individual had exhibited in the past and is thought to still possess. Third, the elderly individual may have possessed the adaptive skills necessary to function quite adequately in their younger years, but physical limitations or accumulated cerebral losses actively inhibit the exhibition of such skills in daily life. Fourth, adaptive behavior may not be exhibited because this behavior, though it existed at one time, has ceased to be followed by contingent reinforcement. Adaptive strategies are subject to extinction just as any behavior. Given the general population's low expectations of elderly persons and the reduction of responsibility which results from institutionalization, the paucity of reinforcement for independent functioning is widespread. As it may be discerned, one's therapeutic approach very much depends upon differentiating these four possibilities with each elderly client.

A simulated role-play situation should help differentiate between skills that are suppressed and skills which are simply not being utilized at present. After rapport is established, and in the absence of negative consequences, the elderly client who shows skills deficits because of anxiety should be able to exhibit adequate skills in this situation. The elderly client who never had learned the skills in the situation or who has lost the competence due to physical involvement will not show these skills regardless of the structure of the interview situation. Gradual shaping through the use of positive reinforcement may reveal behavior which has become extinguished.

Reports from others and a complete social and educational history should supply the necessary information to delineate prior level of competency. If the client could have reasonably been expected to show these skills at one time, given the previous level of functioning, the assessor should begin to differentiate between anxiety-suppressed functioning, loss of functioning due to physical factors, or losses through extinction.

There are several scales which are designed to measure skills level and competency in a variety of situations for use with the elderly. One of which, designed by Salzman, Shader, Kochansky, and Cronin (1972), is intended to measure behavioral changes due to the administration of psychotropic medication with the elderly. It includes fourteen scales concerning a variety of behavioral responses and client abilities. Kastenbaum and Sherwood (1972) utilized the VIRO test to assess the behavior of elderly persons in the interview situation in order to provide additional data, assess treatment outcome, and for screening.

Two other scales were studied by Lawton and Brody (1969) for use with older people. Responses on the Physical Self-Maintenance Scale (PSMS) and the Instrumental Activities-of-Daily-Living Scale (IADL) were compared to, respectively, the ratings of Licensed Practical Nurses and Social Workers' ratings. The RSMS, which assesses skills in the area of toileting, feeding, grooming, dressing, ambulation, and bathing, showed a +.87 inter-rater correlation with the ratings of LPN's. The IADL scale, which assesses competency in the use of a telephone, shopping, food preparation, housekeeping, laundry, transportation, self-medication, and the conducting of finances, yielded an inter-rater reliability coefficient with social worker's ratings of +.85. More importantly, both scales were significantly correlated with behavior and other measures such as physical condition and scores on a mental status questionnaire.

Functional disability measures are also included on the Stockton Geriatric Rating Scale (Meer & Baker, 1966). This 33-item questionnaire was tested on 1381 persons, 65 years of age or older. Communication ability, social behavior and physical limitations are among the skills assessed on a 3-point scale. This scale shows an overall inter-rater reliability of +.87 and a coefficient of internal consistency of +.94. Though this scale is important in the gathering of nomothetic information, it is less useful in specifying individual competency.

More direct measurement of the ability to perform specific tasks while being observed should provide more accurate information with minimal demands. If one desires to measure incontinence, ambulation, or hygiene skills, it is advisable to set up the environment to directly test these skills. Given the data that the elderly often perform poorly in test-taking situations, observation in the natural setting should not only provide more accurate and valid information, but should also result in less anxiety on the part of the client being assessed.

## TARGET BEHAVIOR

The results of the assessment process should ultimately lead to an explicit, quantifiable, and operational statement of the behaviors to modify. This statement of behavioral objectives should take the place of the traditional stage of diagnostic labeling when functional disorders are primarily the target and organic involvement is minimal. Phrasing statements in behavioral terminology aids treatment design and implementation, gives a measure of subsequent progress, gives the client goals and subgoals by which to assess and observe change, and increases the accountability of the procedure and the implementor of the procedure. This latter benefit is discussed by Goldfried and Davison (1976, p. 17).

> We would like to suggest, however, that *the client is never wrong.* If one truly accepts the assumption that behavior is lawful—whether it be deviant or nondeviant—then *any* difficulties occurring during the course of therapy should more appropriately be traced to the therapist's inadequate or incomplete evaluation of the case. We are not implying that this always means the behavior therapist has been incompetent in the way in which he has conceptualized or handled the case. It may very well be that our knowledge of certain problems, or the unavailability of certain concepts, principles, or techniques at this point in the development of the field simply does not provide us with the ability to meet certain types of challenges. We firmly believe, however, that behavior therapy, when viewed as an experimental clinical approach to human difficulties, provides us with the most workable framework within which to expand the effectiveness of the behavior change process.

It's as if these authors were referring specifically to the state of affairs in geriatrics when they mention heretofore unmet challenges and deficits in knowledge.

The target behavior to be changed includes observable, motoric, physiologic "behavior," that which is readily accessible to an observer, and cognitive behavior which is not readily observable but, nonetheless, is amenable to measurement and modification.

The first category of target behavior includes those overt behaviors such as withdrawal and avoidance, chronic complaints, skills deficits or suppression, anxiety, and inactivity. These easily observable behaviors, or behaviors which have observable correlates, may be measured before, during, and after intervention by scales or tests (skills), simple frequency counts (complaints), distance measures (avoidance), physiological indicants (anxiety), or duration counts (inactivity). Scores on self-report measures may augment the total picture since self-report measures offer information of speech behavior.

The second category of targets for change include the cognitive behaviors which can only be assessed through self-report or through some performance measure as on contrived paper-and-pencil tests. Cognitive target behaviors include problem-solving ability, feelings of an external locus-of-control, and inappropriate, negative cognitions. Setting up role-play situations or hypothetical problem situations can result in a direct sampling of the elderly person's cognitive behavior which can then be rated or scored in some manner.

The theoretical bias of such target selection is obvious. The specified targets are all behaviors which, in varying degrees, are observable and/or measurable and require little inferential behavior on the part of the observer. In other words, assessment in geriatric psychology as with any age group is most effective when its subject matter is behavior, not inner-dynamics. In the elderly in particular, assessment procedures which are designed to measure hidden dynamic mechanisms do not yield results which promote economical and effective treatment. Only a functional analysis can be expected to result in such an outcome.

Theoretically, there is no difference in the application of a functional analysis to the problematic target behavior exhibited by elderly clients with that exhibited by younger clients. Regardless of the age

of the client, an assessment which includes concern for the antecedents, consequences, and individual differences of a response, should
prove to be as effective as possible in the solution of those problems
in an area in which our knowledge is still quite limited. A few specific
differences in the application of assessment due to age are discussed
in the next chapter.

# 6
# Special Considerations in Assessment

In the two previous chapters, age-related patterns of responding and some frequently encountered causative variables were described. These considerations are necessary for complete and accurate assessment of geriatric behavior. There are also more specific variations in the process of assessment necessary for interactions with many elderly clients. These variations or supplements are usually necessary because of the differences in functioning of the elderly age group. Some of the more relevant differences which influence the issue of assessment include memory impairment, reduced sensory acuity, lower fatigue threshold, lessened ability to respond to nonconcrete stimuli, and changes in levels of alertness.

In addition to these client characteristics which accompany aging, one needs to include, during the assessment process, stimuli which will elicit the types of information which are particularly relevant to a functional analysis of geriatric behavior (i.e., compensatory behavior, recent relocation, changes in status). Therefore, modifications must be made in two areas, the process of the assessment and the content of the assessment.

The general aim of assessment will become clear throughout this chapter. Assessment should provide specifiable and measurable target behaviors which the client and therapist choose to change. It is important in the design of sound, idiosyncratic treatment plans for the interview, the intake, tests, and behavior sampling, to yield *measurable* targets for change.

## INTERVIEW AND INTAKE

Modifications in the process of the interview which may be dictated by aging correlates include the following:

1. Generally the interview should be shorter than with most age groups as even healthy elderly clients tend to show the effects of fatigue after approximately 40 minutes. Elderly clients with some brain impairment may not attend for longer than 5–10 minutes so the client must be seen repeatedly until sufficient information is gathered.

2. When the elderly client exhibits reduced visual acuity, the interview should be conducted during times when lighting is sufficient. Reduced lighting and contrast when impinging upon less efficient receptors may lead to confusion, slowed reaction times, and errors. Such a result would lead to adverse and atypical responding. In general terms, information should be gathered when the stimulus conditions are optimal so as not to negatively bias the results.

3. Positive reinforcement in the form of verbal encouragement and praise should be randomly delivered by the interviewer in order to increase the quantity of information reported. As cited in the first chapter, increased accuracy in elderly persons' performance is gained by programming positive reinforcement for production. It is important that the reinforcement be delivered randomly, not contingent upon certain types of information (particularly those which may fit the interviewer's orientation or preconceived notions).

4. It is also important to allow sufficient time to respond either to interview questions involving historical information or to test items. Emphasizing speedy response in either circumstance only results in every elderly client looking poorer than daily performance would indicate and, thus, yielding less valuable information. Differential diagnosis is not enhanced by the requirement of speedy response.

5. Supplemental information from other sources should be acquired any time that the veracity of the client's report is suspect. Informal validation for even innocuous responses should be routine since confabulation and denial is often quite difficult to detect during limited contact.

It is usually necessary to ascertain important historical antecedents through the elicitation of observations of others. Family members, relatives, friends, and associates may be able to fill in gaps in remote memory function. Though most historical information does not impact on the present problem since current determinants are most important, earlier psychiatric intervention, educational deficits, and life stresses should be helpful in differentiating between such behavioral manifestations as chronic organic mental disorder, retarded cognitive functioning, and depression.

6. The intake procedure should entail the acquisition of lab work in several areas particularly if the onset of the problematic behavior is acute. Standard tests should include, minimally, glucose levels and electrolyte assays.

Other tests should be requested as needed or indicated by the presence of other clinical symptoms. Practice in geriatric facilities suggests that there are almost no situations where a referral for inappropriate behavior does not result in some type of lab work or measure of vital capacity.

7. The intake report, a sample of which is shown as Figure 6-1, incorporates the standard data found on behavioral intakes such as behavior during the interview and physical appearance, the presenting problem, designated target behaviors, initial treatment plan, prognosis, and additional comments or observations (see, for example, Goldfried & Davison, 1976, pp. 52-53). For use with geriatric clients the intake report should also include the following: the number, type, and quality of social contacts, recent residential relocations, changes in status either through loss of a role or economic changes, and changes in physical condition.

8. The intake report should include data regarding the presence of potentially problematic medications and physical illnesses. An example of a convenient data form is given as Figure 6-2. This form should serve as a guide to insure adequate coverage of most of the endogenous variables which may result in problematic behavior manifestations.

9. The intake report should include, if indicated, the results of a recent general physical examination. Pertinent diagnoses should be summarized in the appropriate blank at the top of the form. The results of hearing and vision tests are also to be included here.

# INTAKE REPORT

Name:                                    Sex:

Date of Birth:                           Date of Interview:

Age:                                     Interviewer:

Place of Birth:                          Pertinent Diagnoses:


Behavior during interview and physical appearance:


Current therapies and medications:


Results of other assessments:


Current environment:


Recent changes in environment and/or role:


Social contacts:


Activity level:


Presenting problem:


Compensatory behavior:


Target behavior:


Treatment plan:


Prognosis:


Comments and additional observations:

**Figure 6-1.  Sample Intake Report for Use with Elderly Clients.**

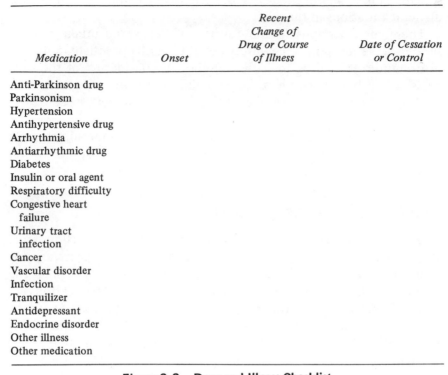

| Medication | Onset | Recent Change of Drug or Course of Illness | Date of Cessation or Control |
|---|---|---|---|
| Anti-Parkinson drug | | | |
| Parkinsonism | | | |
| Hypertension | | | |
| Antihypertensive drug | | | |
| Arrhythmia | | | |
| Antiarrhythmic drug | | | |
| Diabetes | | | |
| Insulin or oral agent | | | |
| Respiratory difficulty | | | |
| Congestive heart failure | | | |
| Urinary tract infection | | | |
| Cancer | | | |
| Vascular disorder | | | |
| Infection | | | |
| Tranquilizer | | | |
| Antidepressant | | | |
| Endocrine disorder | | | |
| Other illness | | | |
| Other medication | | | |

Figure 6-2.  Drug and Illness Checklist.

10. The results from physical, speech, and other adjunctive interventions should be included.

11. The intake report should include observations made of the current living and/or working environments. Pertinent data would include the type of housing, the number of other residents sharing that housing, the adequacy of meal delivery, ease of access to necessary facilities, and a qualitative statement regarding the amount and variety of stimulation present in that environment.

12. The intake report should include data regarding the current activity level of the elderly client particularly any recent changes in the quality or quantity of the activity.

13. Compensatory behavior should also be considered. This section should include other problematic behavior, current personal resources and skills, adaptability of cognitive strategies and problem-

solving ability, and examples of the client's attempts at coping with difficult situations in the past.

These modifications in the format of behavioral intake reports should serve to point the interviewer toward potentially valuable information as well as to more completely consider all of the variables which have been identified as being pertinent to geriatric psychology. The ultimate goal of complete data assessment, of course, is to more adequately develop a plan for treatment.

Another area of assessment which necessitates minor adjustments when dealing with elderly clients is the recording of behavioral samples through naturalistic or contrived observation.

## DIRECT SAMPLING OF BEHAVIOR

Behavior therapists are usually characterized with their clipboards, stop watches, and oddly coded forms. These tools are necessary for sound observations of behavior in those environments in which the client spends his/her time. A strong point of differentiation between behavioral and other approaches has been this desire to obtain a sample of behavior in the environment in which the client is having difficulty. Most behavioral clinicians assume that one's behavior on a standardized test is representative only of that person's behavior in that or similar test situations and not necessarily in the stimulus-response-consequence complex in which the problematic behavior is manifested. It is doubtful that the clinician will be called upon to alter an elderly person's test behavior, per se. Most tests do not adequately represent the situations which they are designed to measure; that is, the situations which may elicit depression, anxiety, coping, and so forth.

For these reasons, it is often valuable if not necessary that the assessor measure behavior in "real-life" situations such as on the ward, in the client's home, or in the presence of those stimuli which result in inadequate responses (Lawton, 1973). Such direct sampling tends to lead to less drastic inferential statements concerning the behavior of interest. It is sufficient, with this methodology, to simply count or score certain responses to naturally occurring, and countable, stimuli. Behavior sampling methodology is well documented elsewhere (e.g., Bijou, Peterson, Harris, Allen, & Johnston, 1969;

Kubany & Sloggett, 1973) and need not be elaborated here. However, there are certain aspects of such sampling which may be differentially affected by age-related variables.

1. Special attention is necessary to insure that the level of arousal of the subject is representative of that client's usual level of arousal. For instance, while observing self-stimulatory behavior in elderly persons, it was noted that at times the frequency of such behavior was atypically low. The resulting bimodal frequency distribution was so striking that further exploration was indicated. Analysis of the observation times showed that these low rates occurred about half an hour after lunch. It became obvious then that, though we were alert enough not to record the subject while asleep, we had failed to consider the decline in activity level between lunch and the time the subject nods off. Some of the positions we had to take relative to the subject being observed resulted in the subject's face and eyes being hidden. It should be sufficient to note that the level of alertness varies and that time intervals should be taken from a diverse number of times of the day.

2. The problem of reactivity during observation is particularly acute with elderly clients because of the paucity of stimuli many of them have in their surroundings. In other words, it is extremely difficult to achieve the optimal situation in which the observer fades into the ongoing background, when there is little ongoing background in which to fade. Though sensory acuity may be so reduced as to make proximity less a problem, it should not be automatically assumed that the observer is not affecting the behavior of his or her client.

3. Though the length of the individual time intervals and the method of calculating frequency and reliability need not be different it may be wise to use shorter but more frequent sessions. This modification helps to eliminate confounds such as lessened arousal and increasing fatigue.

## TESTS, SCALES AND INVENTORIES

It can be briefly and succinctly stated that there are few good tests explicitly designed for use with geriatric clients (Crook, 1979). This state of affairs would not prove devastating except for two major corollaries. First, there are enough significant differences in a variety of areas between elderly and younger test-takers to imply that differences in test design are warranted. Second, since these modifications are not presently available, these tests are being administered to elderly individuals and the results of such tests are not entirely valid. No procedural variance is allowed on standardized tests to accommodate the age-related differences which may affect test performance. Allowing more time to respond, or repeating questions to compensate for these age-differences, of course, would be absurd. One must look elsewhere for the answer other than the modification of test protocol itself.

The clinician may decide that standardized tests which do not have an adequate representation of elderly persons are probably not the most meaningful or useful tests to be administering to the elderly anyway. One's behavior or performance in any area of psychological concern should be judged only in relation to its adequacy in the context in which it occurs (the concept of ecological validity of measuring devices). For example, it is probably not as important for an elderly person in a nursing home to know where rubber comes from (a *WAIS* item) as it is to know how to buy toiletries or where to go to get nourishment. This is not to say that most elderly persons should be concerned only with practical information and not abstract concepts but rather that we, as observers, should not make comments as to level of functioning based upon the amount of useless information which the client has or has not retained. We are no longer interested in making decisions about which classroom the individual would best fit into and, therefore, predictions of future success in academic matters is not as relevant. If we must decide whether a particular elderly client would benefit from a given program, we should observe that client's behavior in activities which share elements of that program.

Most behavioral checklists, surveys, and schedules also do not include items or behaviors which have a high probability of affecting the elderly client. Though assessment devices such as the Fear Survey Schedule, the State-Trait Anxiety Inventory, the Reinforcement Survey Schedule, the Behavior Avoidance Test, and the Beck Depression Inventory are nonspecific enough to be validly applied, the use of such devices with geriatric clients needs some attention. Not only may the process of administration need to be modified somewhat, but most certainly the decisions made based upon the responses on these measures need to include some qualifying statements. For instance, the Beck Depression Inventory contains many items concerning bodily functioning such as changes in appetite, sleep, and sexual interest. It must be remembered that elderly persons tend to show declines in these areas, even in the absence of depression, due to the normal limiting changes brought about through aging. It would also not be unusual to administer the Reinforcement Survey Schedule to an elderly person and conclude from his or her responses that almost nothing appears to serve as a possible reward. But interests also change with age and one cannot expect responses in elderly persons to mirror those of younger persons, or much worse, interpret response differences found in the elderly individual as symptoms of a pathological condition. For example, administration of the aforementioned Reinforcement Survey Schedule (Cautela & Kastenbaum, 1967) should include an appendix with additional items such as shuffleboard, horseshoes, and table games (sports) and crocheting, needlepoint, wood carving, rolling your own cigarettes, time alone, ceramics, Bible study, reality orientation sessions, and crafts (activities).

It should appear clear from the foregoing discussion that new or modified assessment devices need to be established for use with older populations of clients. However, because of the slower response times, the hesitancy to commit responses, and the unfamiliarity with tests and form completion, it may be more advantageous to take a stricter behavioral perspective in assessment. That is, collect data directly from the client and others with regard to the behavior, interests, and abilities of that elderly client. Since it is difficult to argue, especially with older persons, that behavior on a test is representative of behavior on the dimension which the test was designed to measure (and not simply indicative of test-taking behavior), the use of standard techniques should, whenever possible, be minimized.

## ASSESSMENT OF COMPENSATORY BEHAVIOR

The nature and quality of an elderly person's compensatory responses are very important to assessment. Knowledge of this responding helps to differentiate between problems of stimulus control, response efficacy, or response competition.

The main difficulty in this area is the lack of behaviorally oriented, operationally sound measures of compensatory skill. One should hope to strike a balance between the measure of validity and the ability to quantify the data.

Naturalistic observations, which satisfy the first criteria, have typically been subjected to scoring by Q-sort tests while behavior on the Thematic Apperception Test (TAT) has typically been used in an effort to maximize the latter objective. (For an excellent and complete review of assessment of adaptive behavior, see Moos, 1974).

It is, perhaps, more beneficial to discuss compensatory or adaptive behavior, not in terms of coping or cognitive styles, but rather in the quality of an adaptive response in controlled situations. One practical way to do this is to sample the client's verbal report in a variety of situational difficulties and measure the competency of his or her response(s). For example, consider the following potential problem situations and the questions involved:

1. Relocation: "Your physician strongly suggests that you move to a long-term care facility since your physical condition requires continual nursing supervision. How would you handle the news?"

"You have been placed in a nursing home because a new grandchild has been born to your son and daughter-in-law. You want to remain active and sociable. How do you go about fitting into the home? How do you approach your new neighbors?"

2. Limited mobility: "You have recently had a stroke which has left the left side of your body extremely weak. You have to relearn a lot of things that used to come easy to you. How would you go about relearning the necessary skills?"

3. Spouse's death: "Your husband (wife) died two weeks ago. Now that all the family and friends have gone you begin to get an empty ache inside and want to retire to bed all day. How would you combat these feelings of despair? How would you have avoided these feelings in the first place?"

4. Cataracts: "You once were proud of your eyesight, but lately objects have become fuzzy. Your right eye is particularly bad and you are told that there is a cataract there. You are told that you can expect the vision in that eye to get even worse while that in your left eye will gradually worsen, too. What can you do about the prospect? Does the idea of cataract surgery bother you?"

5. Medication compliance: "You were recently prescribed three different medicines which you've never heard of. Your physician tells you their names, when to take them, and what they are prescribed for. You are out of town some months later, however, and you have put the pills in an unmarked container. You're no longer sure which is which or their names. What would you do?"

6. Going places: "You heard that the local library has a fine collection of large-print books but you're not a long-time resident and don't drive. Hou do you go about getting access to these books?"

7. Aging: "A middle-aged friend asks you to give a brief run-down on what it's like to age, any changes, and what you see for the future. What would you tell that friend?"

These sample situations may elicit information about the client's adaptive skills, self-perceptions, views on aging, and the rationality of thought, all of which are valuable data in the assessment process. There are no norms for defining adequate response nor are scoring keys available for the items above. However, the assessor is sampling behavior with regard to response competency which is only a second-level derivative of actual behavior and as such may provide more valid input than responses on a standardized test. Observing actual behavior and rating it as to its adequacy is, of course, the most desirable level of analysis. Whenever possible, the assessor should sample directly the response to similar situations *in vivo*. Responses to these situations, whether the data is verbal report or overt performance, should show how the elderly client is perceiving and adapting to the consequences which often result from correlates of the aging process.

## SOME GENERAL CONSIDERATIONS

Thus far, we have discussed some very specific modifications in the assessment process with elderly clients. These suggestions need not be implemented automatically on contact with every elderly client. However, there are some general considerations which should apply to most interactions. These prompts include the following.

1. A team approach to assessment is most advantageous. Multiple, but unintegrated discipline assessment, at the very least, is requisite. The complicated interrelationships between the variables involved in functional analysis are best considered and evaluated by shared per-

ceptions rather than by one practitioner attempting to assimilate several consult reports.

The multiassessor approach, most often available only in geriatric facilities, should consist of evaluations in the areas of speech, mobility, physical condition, neurology, and pharmacology, as well as psychology.

2. The argument may be made that, if there is a need for a specialized area of psychotherapy for problems of the elderly (i.e., behavioral geriatrics), this specialty should be concerned with assessment, not therapy. Once a decision is made to implement a behavioral or other treatment plan, the modifications in standard procedure are minimal. The attention to many different factors in the assessment process due to the nature of the aged population, however, does suggest peculiar knowledge.

A "specialty" of some superordinate discipline may be defined as one which suggests the need for skills, knowledge, and training different from those of that superordinate discipline and existing specialities. What we are advocating is less a demarcation than an expansion. This breadth may optimally be in the practitioner's skills, but at the least, must involve the practitioner's awareness.

3. The use of single-subject designs which encourage accountability of treatment also aid in the determination of success of assessment. By taking concomitant measures on selected devices, changes in the level of the target behavior may be observed as the treatment is being administered. Taking pre- and postintervention measures over several periods also helps to identify noneffective intervention. If the observed outcome of intervention is unsatisfactory relative to baseline levels, the treatment or assessment may need to be reconsidered. (For a recent survey and description of single case designs, the reader is encouraged to see Hersen and Barlow, 1976.)

Though one typically thinks of these designs as experimental devices, treatment must be just as accountable as research. Particularly in the area of geriatrics where there is so little known and the antecedents are so numerous, constant experimentalism is advantageous.

4. The clinician is constantly faced with the problem of stipulating which area of measurement is of concern in the assessment and

follow-up phases. The notorious lack of concomitant change among the physiological, behavioral (motoric), and self-report indices suggests differing control contingencies.

The clinician then must face the fact that only one of these general modalities or channels of the target behavior (i.e., depression, anxiety) may be affected by the intervention. Which area, then, is to be the criterion for measuring treatment effects? Elderly clients, as would be expected, present no less a dilemma in this regard.

However, one may avoid some of this difficulty if, as mentioned above, a team approach is used. Multiple observers monitoring multiple response channels function almost as a multiple-baseline design. Generally, each representative will be looking at different problematic responses (e.g., cerebrovascular accidents) or the same behavioral complex in different ways (e.g., lack of responsiveness). The benefits are fourfold.

First, the effectiveness of the treatment is evaluated better since the number of observers increases. Second, the likelihood that several response types or modalities are being sampled as part of the improvement criteria increases. Third, the sheer amount of data about the client such as strengths, resources, compensatory ability, historical antecedents and so forth probably increases. Fourth, the client probably will feel that more persons are interested in their case if they have more contact with different people. All of this has, in practice, meant more time spent in evaluation but also more complete treatment planning.

In general, the assessment process should be complete and should incorporate those differential elements which are suggested by the elderly clients' special limitations and situations. The therapist must not be guilty of premature decision-making simply because the client is old or organicity is apparent. We presently have the ability to make accurate differential statements which can result in complete restoration for the elderly client. Though we are quite limited in our ability to reverse deleterious organic processes we have the ability to return many clients to an acceptable level of functioning. Ironically, this recently discovered ability is not due to newly discovered treatment approaches. By reassessing those clients whom we have tagged as "organic" and actively treating their functional problems we can realize a significant gain in the number of successful outcomes. Our future increased success, then, directly results from our assessment errors of the past.

We shall now turn to considerations of treatment with elderly individuals. First, behavioral interventions when organic factors are involved will be discussed. Then, in Chapter 8, behavioral interventions with those problems more often addressed by behavioral therapists are described.

# 7

# Psychotherapeutic Intervention: Organic Mental Disorders

Organic mental disorder (DSM-III) is a catch-all nosological term the use of which strains the validity of classification. When a classification neither suggests an etiology nor a treatment approach, its usefulness is questionable. This was certainly the case with the old label of organic brain syndrome (OBS). Not only may the fixation of a diagnosis of OMD or OBS discourage more active search for specific organic etiology (e.g., site of the lesion, location of the most dramatic atrophy) but it may also prevent active therapeutic intervention. In many cases, OBS leads only to custodial care.

Certainly, there are cases, given large anatomical areas of involvement, poor premorbid resources, and/or long duration of symptoms, where management or custodial care is all that is feasible. This would be the case when and *only when* more active intervention has previously proved to be ineffective. However, given the aforementioned lack of reliability and validity of the classification and the less than absolute assessment process, the diagnosis of OMD should be viewed with some caution.

Often, cognitive changes of any significance initially occurring in the "elderly" years will result in a diagnosis of OMD. If there is no prior history of exposure to mental health intervention, it is automatically assumed that there is an organic cause. The need to specify such cause has typically not been deemed important. Besides this lack of specification, there is a real danger in assuming that age begets organicity and that functional disorders, or the functional consequences of an organically based disorder are unimportant. This chapter is included to explore predominately environmentally based intervention programs. The approach will become obvious, but the philosophy behind the approach should be stressed. No effective intervention program that is currently in practice is aimed at the alleviation of organic mental disorders, per se. As we have seen previously, for practical purposes, there is no such thing as organic mental disorder. The label should act as a convenience *only*. The only valid therapeutic approach involves breaking down the clinical picture of organic mental disorders into the commonly presented problematic behaviors which, when occurring together, often lead to such a diagnosis. There is currently no one panacea which will eradicate this syndrome. First, we shall briefly look at the acute organic behavior changes.

## ACUTE ORGANICALLY CAUSED BEHAVIOR

The techniques for control of problematic behavior secondary to an acute biophysical disorder are as varied as the causes. The elderly client's physician should be called upon to treat the underlying medical problem. This does not mean that the psychologist should stop after assessment. On the contrary, the psychologist's major role now is to make postintervention observations, either through the repeated administration of a mental status evaluation or by naturalistic observation, to insure that the behavioral manifestations are, indeed, becoming less problematic as the medical problem is improving. This practice serves several purposes. First, behavioral indices act as validation that the medical intervention is effective for the targeted etiology. This assumes, of course, that the results of the assessment were initially correct. Second, observation at the overt behavioral level may act as validation that this client is responding idiopathically to the treatment. This assumes that the treatment was correctly administered. Third, this level of observation provides necessary information which helps dictate when the medical intervention, if it is a repetitive procedure, may be terminated. In the case of an electrolyte imbalance causing abnormal behavior, this monitoring may help to prevent "overshooting" the desired level. This assumes that behavioral signs act, at least partially, as the criteria for determining whether or not an elderly client is over the "crisis." The therapist should expect, however, that residual psychological signs may continue to a less intense degree even after the biophysical disorder has been stabilized. Secondary behavioral symptomology may be expected to continue since the negative response to the primary problem and its direct behavioral consequences should not be expected to remit through medical intervention alone. Thus, anxiety will often remain after recovery and may be of such frequency and/or intensity that a psychological therapy for anxiety-reduction may be indicated. Psychotherapy is particularly valuable when the precipitating medical problem may be of a type which can be reinstated by maladaptive behavior (e.g., hypertensive crisis or dyspnea due to anxiety).

Finally, the psychologist may intervene prophylactically by providing the client with appropriate monitoring skills. By learning self-monitoring skills the client may be able to monitor glucose levels, dilantin levels, etc., in order to alert the physician when the levels are beginning to go beyond normal limits. Relaxation training coupled with biofeedback training may help the hypertensive client avoid entering into a hypertensive crisis.

Environmental modifications which may prove helpful *during* the crisis include the following.

1. External stimuli should be carefully regulated such that the client is neither totally inundated with nor deprived of sensory input. It is essential to provide the client with factual data and information regarding their surroundings in order to provide feedback for adequate stimulus control of behavior. This goal may be accomplished by prompting as to date, time, location, names of persons, and objects (reality orientation); keeping the client in a well-lighted and ventilated room with some illumination even at night; keeping outside noise and other noxious stimuli to a minimum; moving slowly around the client; avoiding sudden movements or noises. One quite remarkable clinical observation of behavior secondary to an acute physical disorder involves the patient's response to movement across the visual field. Though often not appropriately responsive to verbal instructions, a startle-type response occurs in the presence of a rapid

movement, followed by an increase in hypermanic motor and/or verbal behavior among many "delirius" clients. If the patient is responding in a depressed manner, the startle response will be followed by further withdrawal. Though it has not yet been empirically established, an additive reaction may ultimately occur which would compound the confusion and further shorten the attention span.

2. A short-term therapy, best described as *distraction,* may be instituted when the client is floridly confused, delusional, or hallucinatory. It is often possible to shift the "delirius" patient's attention to an external stimulus which interrupts ongoing inappropriate behavior. When the stimulus is withdrawn the inappropriate behavior seldom returns immediately. Several such interruptions are usually necessary for cessation of the bizarre behavior. Since the nature of the confusional behavior is not understood, particularly the link between physical upset and behavioral signs, it is difficult to specify the mechanism for this effect. However, distraction theories have been suggested for the efficacy of systematic desensitization, stress inoculation training, and other behavioral therapies with some superficial validity. It may be that selective focusing interrupts some cognitive chain of negative self-statements or that focusing on a neutral or pleasant object or image is incompatible with elevating levels of anxiety.

3. *Supportive* therapy may effect a calming influence on the "delirius" client. The therapist's presence not only serves the function of providing a constant, familiar stimulus, but the therapist's behavior may more directly modify the client's agitation and/or withdrawal through prompts to use relaxation skills or coping statements. Any trained mediator, such as a nursing assistant, aide, or visitor may serve a similar purpose.

Even though the etiology may be biophysical and the antecedent an endogenous one, the behavior therapist has a very important role to play in the treatment of an acute medically caused behavior problem.

## CHRONIC ORGANICALLY CAUSED BEHAVIOR

We shall discuss our therapeutic approach to this frequently encountered area of dysfunction with two concepts in mind. First, problematic behavior may be the consequence of the biophysical etiology itself (the direct result of tissue loss). Second, the indirect consequences which result from stimuli associated either with the organicity itself or other associated variables (e.g., institutionalization, stimulus paucity, expectancy, loss of control) may be present to complicate the picture immensely. It should be noted that the secondary or indirect complicating factors may be, in and of themselves, etiologies of a functional nature. This complexity is noted by Ernst, Beran, Safford, and Kleinhauz (1978, pp. 468–469).

> We propose, therefore, to regard the relationship between the organic structure of the brain and the emotional, cognitive, and behavioral performance of the aging person in a circular model, in which causation may go in either direction. The determining factors are the intervening variables of relative isolation which alter the functioning of the person, produce affective disorders, and disturb cognition. Morphological change alone is not always sufficient unless it is mediated by isolation, and thus results in functional disturbance. Indeed, it is possible that such isolation, as it leads to sensory deprivation, will produce morphological change which in turn will increase the degree of isolation.

In our discussion of the psychotherapeutic approaches to long-term organic disorders we will concentrate, however, on those behaviors which are highly correlated with tissue losses. These behaviors may also be correlated with the results of treatment or individual compensation for functional losses (secondary consequences) which will be discussed in Chapter 8. The behaviors which frequently present with cellular deterioration include disorientation, lowered sensory responsivity, wandering, incontinence, self-stimulation, and inappropriate sexual behavior.

As mentioned in Chapter 3, the behavioral approach to therapy is concerned with the modification of inappropriate behavior, including the behavior mentioned above, through systematic and empirically validated manipulation of functionally related variables. If a client is displaying inappropriate sexual behavior (the response) it may be due to inappropriate stimulus control over that behavior (public display versus private preference), or it may be due to the attention that he or she is receiving for the behavior (positive consequence). If the former proves to be the case, a stimulus control procedure may be implemented, in which positive reinforcement for the sexual behavior is provided only when it occurs in the appropriate place, and aversive stimuli provided when that behavior continues to occur in an undesirable location. If the problem lies in the events which follow the exhibition of that behavior, then those events will be the target of modification such that others who see the inappropriate behavior will ignore (extinguish) the behavior, or punish it. Hopefully, this brief and oversimplified encounter with behavior therapy will serve as an adequate introduction.

## ORIENTATION

As noted in Chapter 4, disorientation is one of the most salient symptoms of organic involvement. Fortunately, determination of the level of orientation can be achieved rather objectively through the client's responses to simple questions. Thus observable targets for change are provided. Disorientation is generally judged to be present when the client fails to respond accurately to questions involving the name of the place where the interview is being conducted, the time of the interview, and/or his or her own name or the name of familiar persons present during the evaluation. This questioning follows only after a medical and social history have been taken and carefully read by the interviewer. Inadequate regard for such information may result in labeling an aphasic client as disoriented since his/her responses may sound peculiar, or in the interviewer expecting that a previously oversedated or "delirius" client should know the present date or location.

The functional significance of orientation to time, place, and person is obvious. One's level of independence is contingent upon accurately processing stimuli which lead to knowing where the client is, who he or she is, and the time of day. As these behaviors become less reliable, the client loses control of many aspects of his or her life (e.g., self-medication, proper nutrition) which, ultimately, leads to loss of control. One treatment approach which was designed specifically for the re-establishment of orienting behavior is called reality orientation.

## Reality Orientation Training

Reality orientation as first described by Folsom (1968), is based upon the assumption that continual, repetitive, reminders, in the form of verbalizations by staff and family, as well as by artificial informational cues in the surroundings, will lead to an increase in orientation in moderately to severely regressed elderly clients (Brook, Degun, & Mather, 1975; Drummond, Kirchoff, & Scarbrough, 1978; Letcher, Peterson, & Scarbrough, 1974). Reality orientation involves two approaches. First, structured classes of from five to ten clients are held several times a week, during which the clients are asked to name common objects, identify colors, and perform other simple tasks. Second, the entire staff or family is trained to interact factually with the client throughout the day. This involves reinforcing the client's accurate orienting statements and correcting the client's inaccurate statements. The entire reality orientation approach stresses keeping the regressed client in contact with the external world as that world is perceived by the majority of the nonimpaired population. The process involves rote learning and assessment of the effectiveness of the intervention involves responses to a questionnaire composed of the training stimuli, themselves.

The application of reality orientation with elderly disoriented clients has been the subject of much research. The findings have been mixed, though generally positively portrayed. The statistics are usually unsophisticated and the dependent measures clinically inappropriate. For example, Hogstel (1979) compared twenty confused elderly patients who received reality orientation with twenty control subjects. All were nursing-home residents. The mean ages for the groups were 80 and 84 years, respectively. After reality orientation therapy was completed, and 18-item questionnaire was administered which *contained the same items as those used in the training sessions.* Despite this rather biased method of defining orientation (as responses to rehearsed and drilled questions), there was no significant difference between the experimental and the control groups' responses on the questionnaire.

Citrin and Dixon (1977) compared twelve institutionalized geriatric patients (mean age = 84) with thirteen similar control subjects (mean age = 83). The experimental group received 24-hour reality orientation and reality orientation class in groups of four or five. The patients in this second group were taught the correct responses to items concerning the day of the week, the date, the weather, etc. The authors used a Reality Orientation Information Sheet (ROIS) and the Geriatric Rating Scale as measures of treatment effectiveness. The ROIS contained items such as, "What is your name?," and "What is the weather?"

The results of this study are typical of the research involving reality orientation. The patients who received the two types of reality orientation did score significantly better on the ROIS. However, there were no differences between the experimental and control groups on the Geriatric Rating Scale. Not only does this study illustrate lack of generalization and questionable clinical validity, but the authors conducted multiple t-tests (which artificially increase one's chances of finding significant results when such results are actually due to chance alone) and still only found statistical differences on the scale containing the training items.

A third study along these same lines was conducted by Barnes (1974). Six elderly patients were seen for 30 minutes, six times a week for six weeks. They received in-class reality orientation in groups of three or four. Effectiveness was measured by observations made by the Nursing Director and a questionnaire. No reliability or validity was established for this questionnaire. Though no significant improvement was revealed by the questionnaire, the Nursing Director did feel that the patients, as a whole, had improved. However, one could list possible alternative explanations for this observed improvement other than that attributable to reality orientation itself. Improvements may have been due simply to an increase in the amount of attention received by the patients, or to the increase in the patient's activity level per se (alternatives offered by the author of the study). Expectancy on the part of the subjects and/or the Nursing Director may also be responsible for the cited improvement.

The major drawback in the research conducted on reality orientation should be reiterated. Increasing the number of one's correct responses to a questionnaire over pretraining levels is of questionable *clinical* significance. It is doubtful that, for clinical purposes, this learning is somehow demonstrative of a return to proper orientation. Are the items learned by repetitive rehearsal during reality orientation actually representative of disorientation? If an individual can tell you the names of common objects after such training, does this mean that this individual is now *oriented*? Theoretically, one can only expect, unless the training is augmented, that significant learning is not taking place. Little generalization to other objects or events can be expected and maintenance of this newly acquired set of responses will probably occur only while that client is confronted by the very same stimuli with which he or she was trained.

Despite this limitation, arguments for the continuance of reality orientation training may be made legitimately if this training could be shown to contribute to other appropriate behaviors (e.g., high staff morale or more positive attitudes toward the elderly) or if reality orientation proved to be superior to other approaches which may have been instituted. Little research has been conducted which addresses these issues though the following studies are of interest.

Smith and Barker (1972) looked at the influence of reality orientation training on the behavior of staff members in a geriatric facility. Using a scale of attitudes (Oberleder Attitude Scale) toward the elderly, ninety-four trainees of varying backgrounds were tested before and after training in the methods of reality orientation. A t-test resulted in a significant difference ($p < .01$) which was not present in a control group of untrained individuals. The change from a pretraining score of 48.5 to a post-training score of 46.1, though, hardly appears significant in any terms except those of a statistical nature. Further research into the benefits on adjunctive measures such as attitude change, morale, and, among the clients themselves, general problem-solving ability, are needed to support or refute the inclusion of reality orientation training in geriatric and long-term care facilities.

The second point, that of reality orientation's relative effectiveness, is explored in a study conducted by MacDonald and Settin (1978). These authors studied thirty institutionalized elderly patients (mean age = 64.4) in which they compared fifteen, fifty-minute sessions of classroom reality orientation with an equal amount of time spent in a sheltered workshop. The latter approach involved the making of children's gifts. This behavior was reinforced through the contingent application of positive reinforcement for production. The reality orientation classes met in groups of five and involved the reading of a reality orientation board which contained facts about time, place, and weather, as well as discussions of news articles.

MacDonald and Settin employed three dependent measures, a Life Satisfaction Scale, ratings by nursing personnel, and behavioral observations.

Only those subjects who were involved in the sheltered workshop showed significant increases on the Life Satisfaction Scale and on one part of the nursing ratings which involved social interest. Not only were there no significant improvements on either measure for the subjects in the reality orientation class, there was actually a slight *decrease* in life satisfaction as measured by the Life Satisfaction Scale.

Thus far, adequate support for the claims of reality orientation proponents has not been established as a recent study by Schwenk (1979) has shown. Though reality orientation is the most widespread nonsomatic attempt to deal with chronic-organically caused behavioral deficits (as well as deficits due to nonorganic etiology), the therapist must not be content to implement reality orientation alone for his/her clients. Behavior theory suggests several modifications and augmentations which may be more beneficial.

## Modified Reality Orientation

One possible approach is to program into the regular reality orientation instruction new methodology which would increase the probability of generalizing therapeutic gains. Enhanced generalization might occur through several means. First, reality orientation items used in the training phase could include information regarding *relevant environmental cues.* Repetition of responses to cues such as the location of rest rooms, stairways, and dining rooms, as well as the names of nursing personnel, the attending physician, and other staff members serves a much more functional purpose and is more likely to be continually reinforced after the training terminates. Second, the problem of questionable clinical validity with traditional reality orientation could be alleviated greatly by teaching skills, not verbal responses which would, in turn, promote generalization and meet with positive results even when situations, physical environments, staff members, familial relationships or other impinging stimuli change. The following case is illustrative.

A seventy-two-year-old male, with a diagnosis of senile dementia secondary to generalized arteriosclerosis, had been involved in

group, individual, and twenty-four-hour reality orientation programs for about two years. Though he appeared to be lucid at
times, this patient could not respond to the typical reality orientation questions a majority of the time (90% of the times tested).
The patient was then trained, by gradual shaping of responses
through positive reinforcement, to identify nursing personnel by
their uniforms, feed himself to verbal prompts involving the major
food groups, and to interact with other patients when the discussion contained personally relevant material. Though his responses
on the typical reality orientation questionnaire did not show great
improvement, he scored significantly higher on a measure of independence in daily living activities and showed no declines when
moved to another floor of the same facility.

The assumption underlying a combined approach is that orientation is not a passive, rote learned set of responses, but rather a
response-complex containing the client and his or her actions upon
the environment. These actions may be seen as adaptive behaviors
which are more appropriate, functional, and ecologically valid than
either the pretreatment response or the responses which are trained
through standard reality orientation. For example, an elderly nursing
home resident may be trained, through conventional reality orientation, to "know" that Tuesday falls between Monday and Wednesday
or that 6:00 p.m. is dinner time. However, these facts alone would
serve little functional value should that client visit the home of a relative for several days. However, teaching the limited geriatric client
how to use a calendar or clock (perhaps using their medication times)
could reduce dependency upon others which would then generalize
to different situations. Teaching compensatory skills to replace those
lost due to organic involvement should provide responses which all
but the most severely cognitively impaired client can learn.

A third way to program-in more valid responses into traditional
reality orientation training would be to gradually expand the level of
material, demands, and tasks within the classroom setting. Instead of
moving a reality orientation "graduate" to a remotivation, resocialization, or attitude therapy group (Barns, Sack, & Shore, 1973), the
judicious use of positive reinforcement (operant conditioning) should
lead to more advanced and appropriate cue-response learning. Moving
from the task of matching colors with fruit, for example, one could

prompt and reinforce correct identifications of colors with wings or floors of the facility; colored name tags with staff duties, or, eventually, times of the day with certain activities of daily living. Throughout training, it is important to provide the chronically impaired individual with responses that are likely to be reinforced naturally by the environment, so that these responses will more likely continue after reality orientation classes are terminated.

Another modification, this concerning outcome research, involves the need for the development of methods which would prove useful in differentiating those clients who would benefit from reality orientation from those who would suffer. It has been this author's experience that some clients would be better served, in terms of freedom from anxiety and depression, by not encouraging them to interact realistically with their current surroundings. At the risk of being labeled pessimistic, one should recognize the fact that certain factors may preclude confrontation with "reality." These factors include:

1. Rapid progression of an illness considered to be terminal.

2. In the very old population, more than two years of total disorientation and social withdrawal where the client lives in what is usually described as "another world." This "other world" actually is the client responding to covert stimuli to which we have no access. Responding to covert, "nonreal" stimuli is evidently serving a compensatory function which probably should not be challenged if the duration of such responding has been lengthy.

3. The presence of intense anxiety or panic when pushed to become oriented to present cues. In psychiatric jargon, "blocking" behavior may serve a compensatory function (i.e., not attending to cues which suggest deterioration) which, when challenged, may present more behavioral problems than those presented before treatment.

A final suggestion for change in research tactics involves validation of reality orientation as an approach. The efficacy of reality orientation with or without the modifications suggested above, should be judged by measures other than those used in the actual process. There is little clinical or ecological validity in proving that a method shows changes in a positive direction *when the method itself is part of the judgment criteria.* At the very least, measures of orientation beyond those involved in the training (for generalization) and which extend temporally beyond termination of training (maintenance) should be included.

Reality orientation was an innovative approach to a previously nontargeted problem and population. Where no other intervention is possible, reality orientation may serve a purpose. However, reality orientation has now taken the place that custodial care had served before the 1960s. That is, a "treatment" approach of less than empirically supported efficacy which, when implemented, may actually be iatrogenic. No other attempts to increase appropriate behavior may be attempted, particularly those approaches which require more staff involvement and special training, as long as reality orientation is handy. This premature complacence could, indeed, be damaging.

## THE EFFECTS OF SENSORY DEPRIVATION

Decreases in sensory acuity and the ability to process incoming information, along with the lack of variable sensation resulting from "treatment" combine to severely deprive the elderly chronic-organic client of necessary stimulation. Research has shown that anatomical structure and optimum behavioral functioning require changes in external stimulation (Diamond, 1978). In fact, Diamond reports evidence which shows that no dramatic changes take place in the brain with aging when, and *only* when, stimulation is maintained. In individuals with *no* noticeable tissue damage sensory deprivation of sufficient duration which involves multiple modalities leads to inappropriate and often bizarre behavior including hallucinations, delusions, depression, hypotension, inappropriate ADH secretion (Oster, 1976a), and mania. When external impoverishment of stimulation occurs on top of an already limited processing system, the problems are exaggerated. It is the effect of sensory deprivation which does the most to confuse the functional-organic differentiation (Ernst, Beran, Safford, & Kleinhauz, 1978). Complicated by long-term deprivation, functional problems or temporary medical problems may mirror chronic changes. Indeed, with a certain amount of deprivation, one may well become chronically impaired regardless of the original etiology. Reversing this trend is theoretically simple, though in practice it is difficult given the predominate therapeutic milieu for clients with diagnoses of organic mental disorder.

Oster (1979, p. 365) has developed an analysis which relates decreased sensory stimulation and physical activity with decreased hypothalamus and pituitary responsivity. Decreases in glandular activity leads, in turn, to a decrease in ACTH production. The causative chain is completed by the work of O'Neill and Calhoun (1975). These authors looked at forty-two nursing home residents (mean age = 84.6). Combining the results of auditory and visual acuity tests with two-point tactile sensitivity to form a composite "sensory loss" score, the authors showed a significant correlation of −.35 with mental status evaluation scores. The picture now can be seen as: Stimulus deprivation and lack of activity leads to decreases in ACTH production and anatomical degeneration which, then, leads to mental impairment.

It appears that not only is sensory stimulation necessary for adequate functioning but that the elderly individual who has been cut off from this stimulation, either due to external or internal factors, creates his or her own stimulation as compensation. In fact, self-stimulation may be the most universal symptom of diffuse, chronic-organic dysfunction. Self-stimulatory behavior will be discussed later in this chapter. First, we will discuss treatment designed to increase activity and sensory stimulation.

Oster (1976) suggests physical and speech therapy to provide stimulation. Providing sensory and physical prosthetic devices in order to magnify interactions with external stimuli should also help.

Second, the importance of environmental contingencies on behavior with which the behavior therapist is particularly familiar, can be used to increase responsivity to external stimulation. Though one study (Jenkins, Felce, Lunt, & Powell, 1977) showed that thirty-eight "senile" residents of two nursing homes could have their level of activity engagement raised by simply providing recreational materials, behavioral technology may enhance this effect. McClannahan and Risley (1975) and Spangler, Edwards, and Risley (1977) showed that prompts increase participation in activities tremendously. During the first phase of the experiment, the subjects were presented with materials though no prompts were given. In the second phase, these materials were also placed in the subjects' hands, but the experimenters prompted these subjects to use the materials. The authors found that the additional verbal prompts were a significant component. In fact, engagement in activity was tripled by providing materials *and* asking the resident to use it, or by demonstrating its use. Simple prompts such as, "Would you like to use this?" and "Do it like this," were effective. Risley and Edwards (1978) report that small door prizes also lead to high levels of participation in activities.

As a pilot of a larger study, Hussian and Lawrence (1981) increased on-task behavior in a nursing-home craft class with chronic disorders by following each 10-second interval in which the subject was appropriately engaged with social reinforcement (e.g., "You're doing a fine job" or "That's it, that's good work."). The activity level increased approximately 65%. Quilitch (1974), studying forty-three regressed patients on a geriatric ward (mean age = 62 years), showed that the offer of prizes, refreshments, and special badges for engaging in purposeful activity increased that activity. Treatment in this study lasted five days a week for thirty-five days, 1½ hours a day.

Jones, Brown, Noah, Atkinson-Jones, and Brezinski (1977) used resident prompters to deliver reinforcement for participation in activities among elderly residents of a mental institution. An increase of 45% over baseline levels of activity was achieved.

An important variation on this theme was utilized in another study. Token reinforcement, which utilizes the same principles as above but is more economical and practical, was also found to be effective in increasing exercise behavior in a population of regressed geriatric patients. Libb and Clements (1969), delivering marbles to four such subjects for exercising on a stationary bicycle, utilized a variable ratio (VR) schedule of reinforcement. The amount of "distance" covered on the apparatus necessary for obtaining a marble would change from one interval to the next. This VR schedule of reinforcement increased the exercise rate by 75% and, as a result, lends further support for operant approaches with the elderly.

Though the nature of the institutionalized geriatric mental patients studied is not detailed, Powell (1974) showed that exercise therapy was successful in the modification of other behavior in the elderly. He compared thirty patients who either received social therapy (arts and crafts, music therapy, games, and social interaction) with those receiving exercise therapy (walking, calisthenics, rhythmic movements). Therapy lasted for twelve weeks, one hour a day, five days a week. The mean age of the subjects was 69.3 years with an average of 24.3 years of hospitalization. The dependent variables included were behavioral and cognitive in nature. The former category included the Nurses Observation Scale for Inpatient Evaluation (NOSIE) and the Geriatric Assessment Scale. The cognitive measures included the Memory-for-Designs, Wechsler Memory Scale and the Raven's Progressive Matrices Test. The exercise group showed significant post-treatment improvement on the Wechsler Memory Scale and the Raven's Test. The social therapy group showed no significant changes on any of the variables. Neither group showed significant changes on the behavioral measures.

Programing access, prompts, models, and contingent positive reinforcement is necessary when dealing with the severely impaired client. With their relatively short attention span, memory deficits, high incidence of disruptive self-contained behavior, and the practical problems which correlate (incontinence), properly applied behavioral technology is the sine qua non of an activity program. As MacDonald (1973) states, encouragement alone is not enough, programed reinforcement is the key.

The second way that the behavior threapist may help deter the effects of sensory deprivation is through the disciplined application of multiple-modality sensory input and the careful regulation of total environments (Cautela, 1972). Entire environments may be modified using behavioral principles in order to minimize the detrimental effects of traditional institutionalization.

Programs designed on an individual basis but with a common theoretical and methodological approach are valuable in preventing many of the negative aspects of organic loss. Programs must be instituted which will be easily maintained by natural processes and contingencies when the program designer and implementer leave.

In small family-care homes or in the home of relatives, the entire housing unit may be redesigned to encourage multiple sensory input. In larger long-term care facilities or geriatric wards, self-contained units should be set aside and continual stimulation provided. Multi-textured and colored walls, a variety of fresh scents, periodic piped-in music, and food which neither looks nor tastes quite the same every day help to keep the senses stimulated. Providing for the inclusion of personal effects and furniture decreases the damaging impact of relocation and subtracts from the usual sterile atmosphere. Continuity within the entire facility is important should the client need to relocate intramurally in order to receive the care provided by a higher level of nursing supervision. Periodic group and individual sensory stimulation sessions are superimposed against this level of routine input. These groups should not provide simply passive stimulation but should require some minimal response from the client which is then to be followed promptly by reinforcement. Too often programs and facilities designed for the elderly chronic client require almost no effort on the part of the client to feed himself, respond appropriately in a group, urinate appropriately, or even arise in the morning. Active interaction in an appropriate manner with stimulating surroundings should lead to preprogramed levels of reinforcement. Without all three elements of the functional relationship, that of stimulus, response, and consequence, we should expect no behavior to be exhibited.

## WANDERING BEHAVIOR

Another behavior which is highly correlated with organic involvement is wandering (Cornbleth, 1977). Any change in physical location which results in a person's inability to return to the point of origin, with or without prosthetic devices, will be the definition of wandering behavior. The functional significance of such behavior involves the safety of the client and the time spent in prevention of injury on the part of staff and family. Commonly, the client who wanders is restrained or sedated sufficiently to interfere with the inappropriate behavior. These two approaches lead to further loss of control, dependence, loss of mobility, and sensory deprivation. A behavioral approach which is being studied presently may offer a more desirable alternative.

To individuals observing wandering behavior, it appears as a purposeless and random activity. External cues giving information as to location appear not to be registering nor to be having a significant impact on the wanderer's behavior. Indeed, when these clients' behavior is arrested, they are unable to verbalize their location nor to independently locate their point of departure. However, a controlled analysis of wandering behavior in elderly clients with diagnoses of cortical atrophy shows that this type of client may, indeed, be aware, at some level, of environmental data. Part of a larger study by Hussian (1980) reported observations of three such residents of a long-term care facility which showed that wandering behavior *does* come under external, environmental control. By studying wandering patterns involving weeks of observation, definite consistent patterns developed.

1. These patients spent consistently more stationary time at points

which could be considered as containing the most information, stimulation, and potential reinforcement. All of these clients tended to stop around other persons or in open rooms where others were located, at windows with exterior views, and at water fountains or untended food trays, in order of frequency. If such points of interest are consistently interruptive of the ongoing wandering, associated artificial stimuli may be constructed to control wandering.

2. By mapping the routes of each wanderer and comparing these maps across time it became apparent that consistent geographic patterns developed within subjects. By placing tracings of several accumulated hours of travel patterns on top of one another, little deviation was found. This held true even *when the subject was taken to a different floor where staff and other patients were all different but the floor plan was identical.* This suggests that, though these subjects are disoriented according to traditional measures and definitions, their behavior is under some component of stimulus control. There was little hesitancy, no obvious puzzlement, and no obvious recognition of the fact that this was not the usual floor with the usual personnel, but the patients continued to spend a disproportionate amount of time near items of reinforcing value.

3. The duration of trips and the distance covered decreased significantly when daily periods of free ambulation were provided. A direct relationship is apparent between time spent in physical restraint and the time subsequently spent in wandering.

These observations, taken together, suggest that a program which does not employ restraints may reduce the wandering behavior since this behavior is obviously not random. It appears that relatively simple cues, in this case architectural, are utilized while more complicated cues, such as associated personnel, distance from the ground, and room numbers, are not being used. Given this information, very simple stimuli in the form of colored arrows were set up strategically in the areas that, during baseline, appeared to be the most traveled by the individual subject. The client was trained to attend to these arrows and to follow them in order to return to his/her room for a preferred reinforcement (food, cigarette, or television time). Other colored stimuli were associated with an aversive event (loud noise). These stimuli were placed at points of potential danger (stairwells) or points of departure from the facility (elevators). Though this study is still in its early stages, it appears that the distance covered and the number of level changes (which could lead to injury since a large thoroughfare is adjacent to the front entrance of this facility) are reduced through such techniques. Providing free ambulatory time periods may also be used to reduce unwanted wandering at a time when observation time may be at a minimum. An indirect consequence of these findings has been the reduction in the time spent in restraints and an increase in ambulation.

## URINARY INCONTINENCE

Incontinence is a major problem in the care of elderly chronically impaired individuals. Though this behavior problem is also present in those clients who are not cerebrally impaired, it is a behavior, or rather a chain of behaviors, which invariably accompanies chronic deterioration and as such will be discussed in this chapter.

Incontinence is probably the rudest reminder that a person has lost or is beginning to lose control over his/her own functions. It connotes dependency, loss of control, and physical decompensation and is associated with unpleasant maintenance, expensive linen bills, and continual decubiti (skin breakdown and lesions). Often, a catheter is used to prevent one or more of these associated problems, but these devices are cumbersome, limit mobility, and encourage infections. If one views incontinence as the end result of a complicated chain of behaviors subject to external modification rather than a result of irreversible decline one can see the usefulness of a behavioral approach to the control of incontinence in geriatric patients.

Due to the variety of causes of incontinence including bladder capacity loss, bladder contractions, loss of feedback, slower ambulation, or the presence of residual urine, Atthowe (1972) suggests using a variety of procedures to eliminate this problem. The author has taken these suggestions and, with a modification of the procedure of Blackman's (1977), has utilized a urinary incontinence program with regressed institutionalized geriatric patients.

Twelve urinary incontinent residents of a long-term care facility were observed for two weeks prior to intervention in order to determine a baseline rate of urinary "accidents." After this baseline phase was completed, the following procedures were implemented by nursing personnel.

1. Assist the resident to the toilet within fifteen minutes of awakening in the morning. If the resident does not void, retoilet every half hour.
2. Offer the resident toileting every hour. Praise him or her if your offer is accepted and then toilet immediately.
3. Praise the resident if he or she voids. Inform the resident if no voiding occurs.
4. After four hours of no voiding, toilet the resident every half hour. (This four-hour limit is most important.)
5. Toilet within fifteen minutes after an accident. An accident includes wet clothes and/or the presence of urine on the bed, floor, or chair.
6. After every toileting, check for wetness of clothing one hour later. Praise the resident if he or she is dry, inform the resident if he or she is wet and have the resident change clothes. If the resident cannot dress him/herself, do so yourself.

This intervention procedure incorporates the elements of stimulus control, feedback, and positive reinforcement contingent upon appropriate voiding. Following two weeks of this intervention, a return-to-baseline phase was introduced in which no reinforcement or feedback was given. Figure 7-1 reveals that a return to the treatment phase after the second baseline period was not necessary. A follow-up phase was conducted two weeks after the baseline was terminated. As can be seen, the number of accidents across subjects declined from an average of thirty-three per day during the first baseline to an average of four at the return-to-baseline phase. It should be noted that only two of the twelve subjects showed any accidental voidings at follow-up.

The control of urinary incontinence in this population is another example of providing strong environmental cues to control an aspect of the activity of the chronically organic client when the internal cues or more subtle external cues cease being influential. The next area of inappropriate behavior sometimes found with this population that will be discussed shows the efficacy of such "supernormal" stimulus control once again.

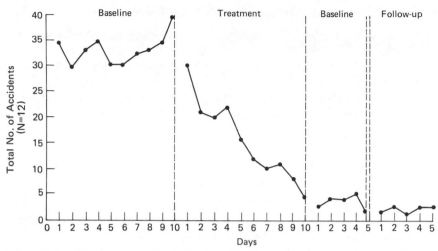

**Figure 7-1.  The Effects of a Behavioral Program on Inappropriate Voiding in Geriatric Patients.**

## INAPPROPRIATE SEXUAL BEHAVIOR

One less frequently observed set of behaviors which correlates moderately with chronic organic deterioration is inappropriate sexual behavior. Though occurring less frequently, the nature of this behavior and the negativistic responses of observers which often follow necessitates attention. Inappropriate sexual behavior often noted with this population includes nonseclusive masturbation, fondling of other patients, and exposure of the genitalia (usually by the male). It is important, for functional reasons, to eliminate this inappropriate behavior.

First, the occurrence of such nonconstructive behavior prevents the programming of more adaptive behavior. Inappropriate sexual behavior occupies a part of the patient's total waking hours, thus preventing such programs as skills training, group sensory stimulation sessions, modified reality orientation training, or bladder control training.

Second, this behavior is particularly bothersome to observers and family members. This point is not meant to indicate some intrinsic negative aspects of the behavior itself, but rather points out pragmatically that the exhibition of such behavior does result in negative consequences for the exhibitor and feelings of uneasiness for most observers. Repeated episodes of such behavior have often led to even more negative behavior on the part of others. Sometimes this includes placement in a mental institution, sedation, restraints, and/or the prevention of participation in therapeutic and social activities for the exhibitor.

Third, this behavior often leads to anxiety and concern among relatives and friends who knew the premorbid behavior of the client. The newly revealed behavior often results in misattribution on their part. Instead of viewing the behavior as a result of decreased inhibitory control secondary to cerebral tissue loss, those close to the client may attribute the sexual behavior to a loss of moral fiber, a revelation of the patient's "true personality," or "father-as-a-dirty-old-man." This may be one instance where the medical model and attributions to tissue pathology is more than welcomed.

The problem with inappropriate sexual behavior in the elderly seems not to fall in the typical schema that is associated with younger "deviants." Typically behavior therapists talk of disorders of arousal or performance. This division covers the traditional fetishes and other socially unacceptable targets as well as impotency, frigidity, and vaginismus. In the elderly chronically impaired patient, the problem is more a loss of appropriate control, within the environmental context, than a qualitative difference in the response or the target. Often, once we escape the chronological biases that we may possess, the behavior that we see appears bizarre and inappropriate *only in the setting in which it occurs*. If for no other reason than that it is probably none of the therapist's business, the situation and setting for the behavior should be the target for change, not the response itself. In geriatric and long-term care facilities there are old homosexuals, old nymphomaniacs, and old "philiacs" of all types, just as there are in any group of people (e.g., hospitals, dormitories, conventions). Time is more optimally spent in training the behavior to occur with a higher probability in a setting which would minimize the problems mentioned above. Karoly (1975, p. 215) presents this view.

In many therapeutic situations, it is easier, cheaper, or faster to program antecedent stimuli for appropriate responding than to try to identify and alter the contingencies. And . . . not all clinical problems require behavior acceleration or deceleration—but rather responding in the right place and at the right time (stimulus control development).

Building appropriate stimulus control of inappropriate sexual behavior in these patients requires more time, more salient situational cues, more continual reinforcement, and more booster sessions than with a population of intact individuals. Due to some of the reasons cited in Chapter 1 concerning the changes in normal aging as well as the changes noted in Chapter 4 surrounding chronic organic impairment, these extra efforts are understandable. Still, the process of therapy is basically the same. The therapist designates one area and/or one time in which the client's behavior is considered appropriate, meaning that it will be followed by a positive event. All other times and places are considered inappropriate for that behavior while being appropriate for other responses. One then, after collecting baseline observations, teaches the person to discriminate between these two locations (the appropriate place to engage in sexual behavior and all other places) by selectively reinforcing differential behavior in these two areas. This process is called behavioral engineering. The following case should illustrate this procedure.

A sixty-two year-old man in a moderately sized nursing home was referred for frequent masturbation in front of the nursing desk and in resident lounge areas. This resident had no history of sexual inappropriateness or dysfunction. The employees of the home and family members were quite embarrassed and repulsed by this behavior. The resident was labeled as a "pervert" and a "mental case" by a majority of the staff. He did not respond to reprimands or rule-setting.

Baseline data, including the frequency of masturbation behavior, location of the behavior, time of occurrence, immediate consequences, and others present, were collected by nursing personnel for two weeks. It became clear on examining these data that the behavior occurred independently of context (setting, consequences, the reactions of others, etc.). Therefore, a stimulus control procedure was begun to make the behavior likely to occur only in the resident's room, with the curtain drawn, the door closed, and the roommate out. Staff members were instructed to terminate the masturbatory behavior after it began but prior to ejaculation by grabbing the resident's hand and leading him to his room. There he was allowed to continue masturbation only when he completed the behavior which would meet the criteria above (i.e., making sure that the roommate was gone, closing the door, closing the curtain). Initially, a large orange disc was placed on the wall above his bed and in his bathroom which acted as a cue in the presence of which masturbation was permitted. Masturbatory behavior occurring wherever this artificial stimulus (artificial meaning not inherent to the usual context) was not present was interrupted. This procedure may be considered by some to be punishment though prevention of a pleasurable event contingent upon an inappropriate behavior is, by definition, negative punishment or extinction.

The behavior quickly became specific to the appropriate stimuli (the room and orange disc) such that, after six days of this treatment, every incident of sexual behavior occurred in the privacy of his own room. From an average of almost eight incidences a week, there were no further public displays even at a two-month follow-up. The orange disc was made smaller and smaller, gradually fading, in four steps, until it was no longer needed. The masturbatory behavior had come under the control of the room, not the artificial stimulus.

Stimulus control of sexual behavior is a very effective procedure except in cases of postcerebrovascular accidents. Stimulus control may not be effective in these cases since the functional analysis of the problem behavior should reveal a deficit in muscular control rather than in stimulus control. Spastic limb movements and loss of even gross motor coordination may result in behavior which, topographically, resembles fondling, hitting, or patting. Neither the patient, the patient's family, nor the staff benefit from continuance of the belief that the behavior is volitional. Simple advice to the contrary is often all that is needed. It is also possible that repetitive contacts between the genitals and other parts of a client's body are more appropriately viewed as the self-stimulatory or stereotypical behavior of a nonsexual nature often seen in this population.

## SELF-STIMULATORY BEHAVIOR

This is the final set of behaviors to be discussed in this chapter though it appears last not because of a lack of frequency or importance. On the contrary, it may be that self-stimulation is the most frequently observed behavior in this group and it, in part because of this high frequency, may be the most important. The reason this section is last is simply that less research and documentation of this behavior is available so the discussion which follows may be considered to have less validation than those above.

During unstructured observations of cortical atrophy cases this author noted the remarkable universality of a type of behavior which is marked by its apparent lack of functional utility, its repetitiveness, and its diagnostic-predictive ability. Particularly, when such a patient is partially restrained or his or her movements are somehow limited, these behaviors may continue almost without rest for hours until a distractor stimulus is presented. Self-stimulatory behavior may include rubbing of the palm over parts of the body, a "sanding" behavior of the palm across flat surfaces, repetitive nonsensical vocalizations, picking at the skin or clothes, taking footwear on and off, and the manipulation of nearby objects. This behavior appears to be similar to that displayed by genuinely autistic children or the severely retarded and a possible explanation for its existence may come from research in that area. It is possible that the elderly chronically impaired patient, cut off from external stimuli, is generating his or her own stimulation which serves as sensory reinforcement which, in turn, leads to a continuance of the behavior. Without the ability to process incoming environmental stimulation this patient must resort to self-contained input and the sensory reinforcement which results. If it is true that man requires a certain level of stimulation to survive then the functional significance of this self-stimulatory behavior becomes clear.

A study by Hussian and Hill (1980) is the first attempt to assess the parameters of stereotypical behavior in the elderly client. By making naturalistic observations of four long-term care patients with diagnoses of organic mental disorder, these authors showed that 87% of the time not spent eating or sleeping is spent in this behavior (see Figures 7-2 through 7-5). The study was conducted using a time-sampling method of observation with ten-second observation inter-

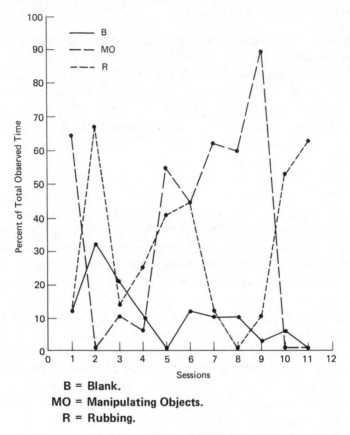

**Figure 7-2.  Subject No. 1.**

**Figures 7-2, 7-3, 7-4, and 7-5.  Amount of Time Spent in Self-Stimulatory Behavior.**

vals interspersed with two seconds of recording and orienting on the part of the observers. Preliminary studies indicate that, barring limb restraints and gags, the only thing that will interrupt this ongoing behavior appears to be the application of a distractive auditory, visual, or tactile stimulus. When this noncontingent external stimulus is removed, the self-stimulatory behavior returns after several seconds. It is hypothesized that ongoing stimulation and fewer restraints to motility should decrease this behavior.

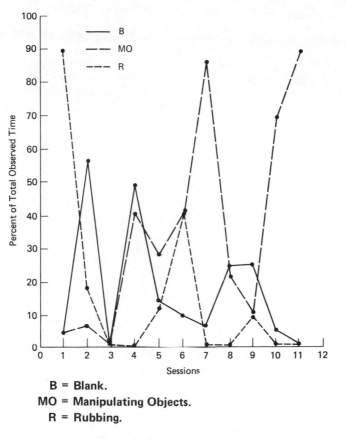

B = Blank.
MO = Manipulating Objects.
R = Rubbing.

Figure 7-3.    Subject No. 2.

A second phase of the first study by Hussian and Hill (1980) provides some evidence as to the predictive properties of this behavior. The second author, an undergraduate psychology minor with no diagnostic experience and blind to the sample composition, was shown twenty-six randomly selected geriatric patients from a 120-bed nursing home. She was not told how many of the subjects, if any, were diagnosed as having progressive cortical atrophy. After less than one minute of observation of each patient, she correctly identified the thirteen patients with diagnoses of organic mental dis-

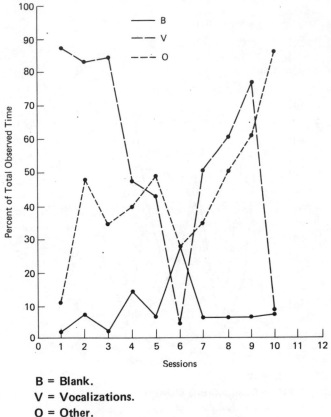

B = Blank.
V = Vocalizations.
O = Other.

Figure 7-4.   Subject No. 3.

order and did not identify any of the other non-brain-disordered patients as having stereotypical behavior.

Self-stimulatory behavior, then, may be useful in the diagnosis of global tissue loss of this sort. It is an area of correlated behavior which deserves additional attention. Along with the other behavioral problems discussed above, the symptom complex of OMD may be attacked, one symptom at a time, in an effort to temper the disturbing prognosis brought on by a chronic organic etiology. It should be emphasized before leaving the problem of organicity that in no other population of this size will the interaction between functional and physical causation and functional and medical intervention be so

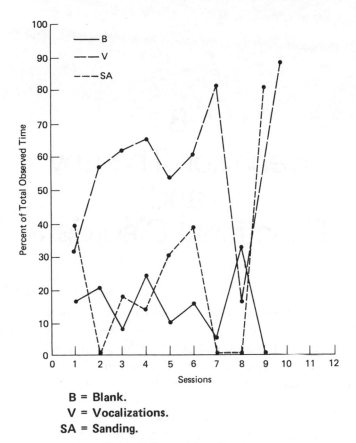

B = Blank.
V = Vocalizations.
SA = Sanding.

Figure 7-5.    Subject No. 4.

important. The foremost challenge in dealing with these clients has always been not to be content with relegating such patients to back wards. Now the challenge is to find new, innovative treatment techniques based upon our newfound optimism.

# 8
# Behavior Therapy
# and
# Functional Disorders

Problems of predominately a functional origin require little approach-modification on the part of the therapist regardless of the client's age. If, after employing the suggested procedural modifications during assessment, organic interactions are minimal, the therapist may, for the most part, proceed as usual. However, some of the qualitative changes which accompany aging, as well as the target behaviors which are mainly age-related, do dictate treatment modifications. We shall again use the general target areas of response competency, response incompatibility, and, to a lesser extent, stimulus control. Some of the behaviors to be modified and the various behavioral techniques may, of course, overlap categories.

## RESPONSE COMPETENCY

There are a variety of behavioral techniques designed to enhance appropriate response. Most of these techniques have survived the test of formal validation (outcome research) as well as less rigorous evaluations (repeated clinical success) in nonsenescent populations. Recently, some of these techniques have been applied to elderly clients who exhibit problems in response efficiency with similarly positive results. These techniques range in theoretical composition from operant conditioning of physical maintenance skills to generalized response-strategy training.

## Skills Training

The training or retraining of skills covers a wide variety of response areas and a wide variety of levels of functioning. Typically, when previously adequate response in the areas of self-feeding, toileting, ambulation, etc., has decreased to near zero rates it is due to extinction and the provisions of others. Responses which are no longer expected to be present tend not to be reinforced by others and even may be prevented from occurring through premature intervention. What then becomes expected and reinforced is a lower level of response from the elderly client. Attempts to re-establish previous levels of response involve the reinforcement of gradually increasing self-management behavior across a variety of areas.

Self-feeding skills were targeted for improvement by Risley and Edwards (1978) in a sample of elderly nursing home residents. Providing adequate nutrition is a common problem among fairly disabled elderly individuals and self-feeding, wherever possible, is a valid goal since aide time may be limited and self-feeding would contribute to increased self-determination. Through a combination of guidance and praise for successive self-feeding attempts, Risley and Edwards were successful in re-establishing self-feeding in a relatively short time. Figure 8–1 shows the improvement over four and two successive meals for three elderly nursing home residents. Guided participation which is gradually faded into self-directed motion with contingent positive reinforcement (praise and the food consumed) combine to increase response adequacy.

Receiving a personally chosen gift contingent upon adequate feeding behavior was found to be successful in a study of six elderly individuals by Geiger and Johnson (1974). These authors found that the percent of their population who exhibited correct eating behavior was 12% before the contingent reinforcement program and 84% after intervention.

Rinke, Williams, Lloyd, and Smith-Scott (1978) utilized prompts and reinforcement in the form of praise, visual feedback, and desired

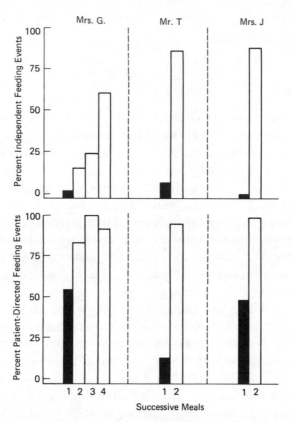

**Figure 8-1.  Level of Independence and Participation Shown by Nursing Home Residents Across Successive Meals when Assisted by Aides using Regular Nursing Home Procedures (dark bars) and the Rehabilitative Feeding Assistance Routine (white bars). (From Risley, T. R., and Edwards, K. A., 1978. Paper presented at the Nova Behavioral Conference on Aging, Port St. Lucie, Florida)**

food items, to promote self-bathing in six elderly nursing home residents with diagnoses of "chronic brain syndrome."

The ambulatory status of two residents of a nursing home, aged 92 and 85, were studied by MacDonald and Butler (1974). These two residents moved throughout the facility in wheelchairs though, physically, there was no reason for them not to ambulate independently. A reversal design was used to check the effectiveness of a contingency intervention in which verbal and nonverbal prompts were used and reinforcement was delivered contingent upon ambulation. Data were recorded in a baseline, contingency, reversal, and return-to-contingency design. The two graphs, Figures 8–2 and 8–3, clearly show the effectiveness of the procedures. Simply interacting in a positive manner with such patients when they are not in contact with their wheelchairs and ignoring their wheelchair behavior, dramatically increased the former more appropriate behavior.

Nonambulation is a particularly frequent problem on the floors of geriatric facilities. A minor injury such as a broken bone due to a fall may result in temporary placement in a wheelchair. The effortlessness of this new mode of transport, coupled with the increased attention the new posture brings from others, may often provide stronger rewards than did ambulation. Strong encouragement in the form of verbal prompts and selective reinforcement for out-of-seat behavior must be implemented in order to return the client to preinjury levels of independent ambulation or ambulation with minimal assistance.

Verbal skills and the appropriateness of verbal behavior have also been targets of change by behavioral researchers. Many of these attempts have dealt not only with verbal behavior per se, but also resocialization through appropriate verbal communicatory skills. Hoyer (1973), Hoyer, Kafer, Simpson, and Hoyer (1974), Linski, Howe, and Pinkston (1975), and MacDonald (1978) have shown the effectiveness of behavioral techniques in the re-establishment of verbal behavior in elderly samples. In these studies, verbal prompts were given as stimuli for elderly subjects to engage in verbal behavior, which, in turn, resulted in the application of positive reinforcement for responding. In the Hoyer, Kafer, Simpson, and Hoyer (1974) study, pennies were given as reinforcers to four nonverbal elderly mental patients. Sessions were held twice a week for an average of fifty minutes. The application of these tokens increased verbal behavior and may, as the authors point out, be easily carried out by paraprofessionals such as nursing personnel.

MacDonald (1978) used an A–B–A–B reversal design with three nursing home residents. By making time-sampling observations of verbal behavior, she showed that social reinforcement and prompts successfully increased responding in these subjects. This time-sampling methodology yielded an inter-rater reliability of .94 thus suggesting the validity of the measurement device.

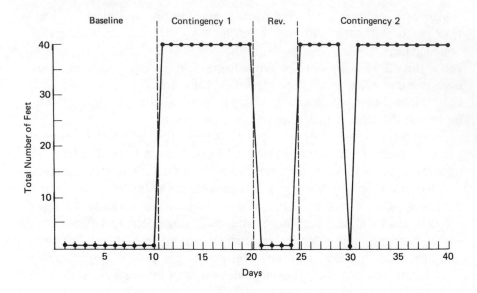

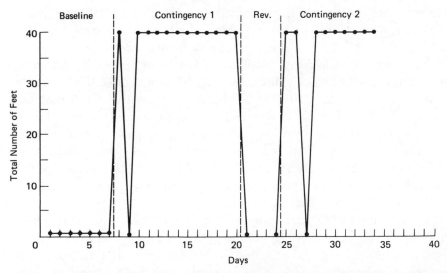

Figures 8–2 and 8–3.  The Total Number of Feet Walked by Subjects 1 and 2 on Each Day During Successive Conditions. (From MacDonald and Butler, 1974, p. 99)

Wisocki and Mosher (1980, in press) have shown the effectiveness of sign language training in an aphasic eighty-one-year-old man diagnosed as a "catatonic schizophrenic." The use of a peer in the training program enhanced the expression of these learned signs as well as other behaviors which correlate with socialization. Figures 8–4 and 8–5 show the effectiveness of prompts, contingent reinforcement and modeling.

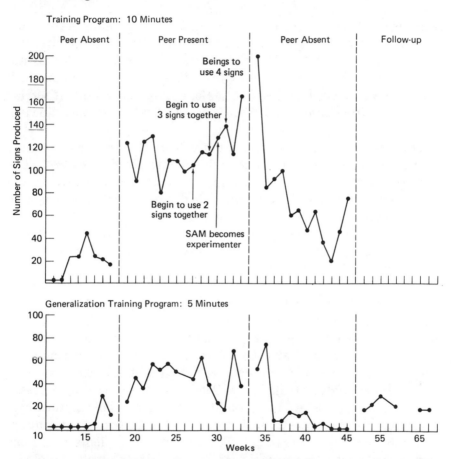

Figures 8–4 and 8–5.  Mean Number of Times Signs were Expressed by Subject under Two Experimental Conditions During Times Corresponding to Peer Inclusion and Exclusion. (From Wisocki, P. A., and Mosher, P. Peer-facilitated sign language training for a geriatric stroke victim with chronic brain damage. *Journal of Geriatric Psychiatry*, 1980, 13, p. 96)

The reinstatement of verbal behavior leads to efforts designed to shape that verbal behavior into a response in social situations. This so-called "resocialization" has been targeted by several behavior researchers. In a study reported by Risley and Edwards (1978), verbal interaction during dining by elderly nursing home residents increased through the simple manipulation of table size. In fact, the number of verbal interactions doubled when the table size was reduced from ten to twelve seats to four to six. Another study also reported in the same paper found that at a typical institutional dining setting, the highest percentage of social interaction occurring during baseline observations was 15.6%. The researchers then compared this institutional style seating arrangement with a family-style situation in which the food was passed around the table, each elderly resident serving him/herself from common dishes. These authors report the following.

Percentages of social interaction for 9 of the 16 residents more than doubled, and only one resident interacted less (1%) when served family-style. Conversational content was primarily related to food in both situations, but when meals were served family-style even non-food-related conversation increased 66%. In addition, during family-style meals individual residents contributed more equally to the conversation than when served institutional-style meals. (Risley & Edwards, 1978, p. 11)

Mueller and Atlas (1972) utilized a group setting with five elderly residents who had low baseline levels of socialization. Through carefully programmed token reinforcement for appropriate interactions these subjects (mean age = 70) showed an increase in the mean number of responses from .85 per half hour session to 5.88 per session.

In another study, Abrahams, Wallach, and Divens (1979) increased social interactions as well as mobility, while decreasing daytime napping and confinement through the use of high school students as "remotivators and socializers." Twelve geriatric patients in a long-term care facility (mean age = 73.2) met with the high school students for fifteen weeks, each session lasting sixty minutes two times a week. Various behaviors were measured on the Sickness Impact Profile. The sessions included verbal interactions, sharing ideas, songs, and parties. In addition to the changes mentioned above, the elderly patients maintained these gains even when the students were not present, thus providing one of the few examples of the application of a successful technique resulting in generalization to other situations.

Interpersonal skill- or social skills-training has been attempted with older adults who are fairly intact cognitively. For example, Berger and Rose (1977) assigned twenty-five elderly nursing home residents (mean age = 77) into either a skills training group, a discussion control or an assessment-only control group. The patients receiving the skills training received three forty-five-minute to one hour sessions with the following training sequence: situation presentation, coaching, modeling, discussion, rehearsal, and feedback using actual role-played social situations. The patients in the discussion control group were presented with the same social situations but simply *discussed* similar experiences. Berger and Rose administered the Interpersonal Situation Inventory (ISI) and the Behavior Roleplay Test (BRT) and a simulated test of "real life" situations. The groups differed at post-test only on the behavioral measure (BRT) with those patients receiving the skill-training performing significantly better than either of the control conditions.

It is significant that such a training procedure effectively improved the training group's performance in interpersonal situations, however the lack of generalizability to new, nontrained, situations is disappointing. This lack of generalizability, which is a common finding in treatment outcome studies with elderly subjects, is not surprising however, since no attempt was made to actively program variables which could enhance this generalization. As the authors point out, the use of multiple models, group format, additional rehearsal, booster sessions, and the encouragement of continued reinforcement from the staff for the newly acquired behavior would help to insure generalizability and maintenance of treatment gains. Social skills, just like any form of behavior, are subject to extinction if they are exhibited without being followed by positive events.

Toseland and Rose (1978) attempted to compare several methods each of which is designed to increase social skills of the elderly person. These authors compared the effectiveness of a behavioral role play approach with a problem-solving training approach and a social group work approach with fifty-three subjects, all 55 years and older. The subjects met in five groups of from three to five subjects for six, ninety-minute sessions. The role play group received training in a manner similar to the Berger and Rose (1977) group who received interpersonal skills training. The problem-solving training group received the traditional Goldfried and D'Zurilla training which includes the problem-solving orientation, defining the problem, the generation of alternative solutions, decision-making, and the implementation of the chosen strategy. The social group work approach involved discussions, in the group, of the best responses to a given situation and a common discussion of the solution chosen.

A role play test and two self-report inventories served as dependent measures of treatment effectiveness. It was found that, on posttest, both the behavior role-play subjects and those who received the problem-solving training showed improved social skills over the social group work subjects on the behavioral measure (see Table 8–1). There were no differences between the role play or problem-solving groups, no differences among the three treatment groups on the self-report inventories (probably due to the ambiguity of the items), nor any significant differences at a three-month follow-up.

Table 8–1   Results of the One Tailed Planned Comparisons for the Role Play Test Trained and Untrained Situations from Pre- to Postassessment and from Pre- to Followup Assessment

| Planned Comparison | Role Play Test Situations | | | |
|---|---|---|---|---|
| | Trained Situations | | Untrained Situations | |
| | Pre-Post | Pre-Followup | Pre-Post | Pre-Followup |
| Role Play Vs. Social Group Work | $4.01^{xx}$ | 1.18 | $4.63^{xx}$ | .86 |
| Role Play Vs. Problem Solving | 1.23 | .47 | 1.07 | .89 |
| Problem Solving Vs. Social Group Work | $2.78^{x}$ | .72 | $3.56^{x}$ | .33 |

[xx]significant at $P < .005$
[x]significant at $P < .01$
From: Toseland and Rose, *Social Work Research Abstracts*, 1978, p. 13.

An informal observation made by the authors is of significance here. They found that those subjects who received the behavioral role play training method expressed the fact that they found that they could handle themselves better in nontrained situations. It is clear that, as in the research with reality orientation, more formal tests of performance on nontraining stimuli are essential to determine generalization.

From physical maintenance skills such as feeding, ambulation, verbalization and continence (discussed in Chapter 7) we have progressed to resocialization and interpersonal skills training. In the research describing such training procedures it is clear that response skills can be increased in elderly subjects. The combination of reinforced practice, shaping, and modeling, have been shown to be effective. However, it should also be noted that, without special attention to ongoing environmental determinants of behavior, these gains have little chance of being maintained.

## Strategy Training

Two other response areas which have been studied include coping with memory problems and cognitive strategy training. Given the age-related differences in these two areas and the negative adaptations which often result from such deficiencies, intervention at this level may alleviate poor compensation as well as reducing responses which are incompatible with compensation.

Zarit (1979) found that the primary memory ability is about the same in elderly individuals and younger subjects but that problems in acquisition and recall are more frequent in secondary memory with elderly subjects. This age decrement is present unless the amount of the material which is acquired is the same for the different age groups. Zarit feels that these age-related deficits are not always due to organic factors and that the teaching of recall strategies or interpersonal skills should erase these age differences and lower the depressive response which often accompanies realizations that the memory is no longer functioning maximally. Zarit found, indeed, that training of recall strategies did increase memory functioning. Labouvie-Vief and Gonda (1976) attempted to train cognitive strategy to increase intellectual performance in sixty noninstitutionalized elderly subjects (mean age = 76). The authors compared cognitive training (self-instructional), anxiety training (self-instructions and coping oriented), unspecifiable (subject's own coping strategies), and no training. The dependent variables included the training task and a transfer task on the Raven's Matrices immediately after training and two weeks later.

On the training task, immediately following the intervention, the cognitive and anxiety training groups showed better performance while on the delayed testing, those receiving anxiety training and unspecified training performed better than the cognitively trained or no training groups. On the test for generalization immediately following intervention, the unspecified group proved to be superior to the other conditions while two weeks later those subjects receiving this unspecific training and the cognitive training performed better than the other two conditions. It seems, therefore, that specific coping strategies are helpful on the training task, but that teaching generalized subjective strategies may be superior for transfer to other tasks involving similar abilities.

Self-instructional and problem-solving training are two behavioral approaches which are designed to improve one's overall coping ability or to guide performance in various task-related or problem situations. Though these methods are also used to reduce inappropriate response prior to response competency building, two examples of the application of these two approaches as response builders are illustrative.

A seventy-nine-year-old woman was self-referred for gradual memory decline. She would find herself half-way to a shopping mall or downtown and forget why she had left home. She was also requiring police aid for walking against pedestrian right-of-way lights at intersections. She was beginning to avoid any contact with the outside, preferring to have neighbors and friends shop for her and run her errands. The therapist set up a program in which a typical trip downtown was mapped out with all stoplights, crosswalks, decision points, and potential problem areas. Timetables, goals, and paths were decided upon with the client. Self-instructions, tied to the cues and stimuli which are necessary for safe functioning were rehearsed. These statements included, "This is the one intersection which I can cross diagonally because of the one-way street," and "I'll go into one of the shops along the way whenever

I forget all five of the items which I came for and refer to my list."
Self-reinforcing statements were programmed to occur at certain
geographic points or at certain points in the written routine. The
client performed well, and despite one neglected item on the first
trip after intervention, had no further problems on subsequent
trips.

An eighty-one-year-old woman, a resident in a long-term care facility with diagnoses of arteriosclerotic heart disease complained of
not being able to make any "real" decisions and periodic feelings
of being overwhelmed and wanting to give up. There were no
immediate practical alternative placements for this client nor was
the entire environment modifiable to an extent sufficient to have
a positive impact on her behavior. Problem-solving training was
begun so as to enhance response competency in the face of unal-
terable environmental contingencies. During the definition-of-
problem stage she pointed to several problem areas such as giving
up her home, relative's fighting over her belongings, and relatives
who visit but disrupt her medical regimen or the ongoing activities
of the staff. Through the training she came to be able to pick solutions, weigh them, and practice them in real life. Her self-reported
general anxiety level was reduced, she reported being happier and
more satisfied, and she eventually sought, and found, more appropriate housing in the community which encourages independent
behavior.

The building of appropriate, flexible responses which are general
enough to be successful in a variety of stimulus situations and which
can be continually followed by reinforcing consequences is extremely
valuable in geriatric psychology. The stimulus conditions which are
specific to aging such as reduced mobility, loss of independence, and
reduced system functioning, may be compensated for by training
skills, approach tactics, and general problem-solving strategies. When
the ability to respond is thought to be present but is not actively
being exhibited, different approaches are needed to reduce or eliminate the behavior which is preventing the adaptive response from
occurring before training more appropriate responses. Some of these
techniques result in the reduction of the problematic behavior only

while others remove the incompatible response at the same time new response strategies are taught which may be directly applied in future situations.

## REMOVING INAPPROPRIATE RESPONDING

A variety of incompatible responses interfere with the elderly client's ability to respond adequately to a variety of stimuli in their lives. The most frequent incompatible response by far is depression (Gurland, 1976). A number of approaches are available to reduce depression, but problem-solving appears, at least on the surface, to have the components necessary for generalization across situations and maintenance across time, more than approaches such as reinforcement for activity or increasing the number of available reinforcers. A study by Hussian and Lawrence (1981) shows the relative effectiveness of such an approach over a purely activity-reinforcement approach.

Thirty-six depressed nursing home patients over sixty years of age were divided into two experimental groups to test the relative effectiveness of a reinforcement approach and a problem-solving approach to reduce geriatric depression. Twelve subjects received social reinforcement for their participation in an activity, twelve subjects received problem-solving training, and twelve subjects served as a waiting-list control condition. During the second treatment week, the subjects were then randomly divided into the following conditions: problem-solving to problem-solving (PS-PS), problem-solving to social reinforcement (PS-SR), social reinforcement to social reinforcement (SR-SR), social reinforcement to problem-solving (SR-PS), waiting-list control to waiting-list control (WLC-WLC), and waiting-list control to an information control (WLC-IC). The Beck Depression Inventory, a self-rating scale (SRS), and the Hospital Adjustment Scale (HAS) were administered to the subjects.

The results can be seen in Table 8-2 and Figures 8-6, 8-7, and 8-8. After the initial treatment week, the two experimental conditions (PS and SR) showed significantly lower Beck and SRS scores than the waiting-list control (WLC). After the random division of the groups (treatment week two) when compared with the waiting-list controls only those groups which received problem-solving training significantly reduced their scores on the Beck. At the two follow-ups,

Table 8-2  Group Difference Scores for Each Dependent Variable.

| Analysis | Condition | Beck | SRS | HAS[a] |
|---|---|---|---|---|
| Treatment | PS | 6.58 | 2.39 | −1.08 |
| Week One– | SR | 5.42 | 2.08 | −1.00 |
| Baseline | WLC | 0.50 | 0.56 | −0.83 |
| Baseline– | PS–PS | 10.17 | 4.33 | −2.00 |
| Treatment | PS–SR | 12.17 | 1.50 | −2.83 |
| Week Two | SR–SR | 7.33 | 0.78 | −0.67 |
| | SR–PS | 10.33 | 4.39 | −1.00 |
| | WLC–WLC | 2.67 | 0.72 | −0.67 |
| | WLC–IC | 1.17 | 0.72 | 0.00 |
| Treatment | PS–PS | 4.17 | 0.90 | −2.00 |
| Week One– | PS–SR | 5.00 | −0.67 | −0.67 |
| Treatment | SR–SR | 2.67 | −0.72 | 0.67 |
| Week Two | SR–PS | 4.17 | 1.72 | −0.33 |
| | WLC–WLC | 1.17 | −0.17 | 1.17 |
| | WLC–IC | 1.67 | 0.50 | 0.17 |
| Follow-up 1 | PS–PS | 11.16 | 4.44 | −3.33 |
| (Two weeks) | PS–SR | 12.20 | 1.13 | −1.00 |
| | SR–SR | 2.20 | 0.73 | −0.40 |
| | SR–PS | 10.00 | 3.67 | −0.80 |
| | WLC–WLC | −0.16 | 0.05 | 0.33 |
| | WLC–IC | 2.66 | 1.78 | −1.17 |
| Follow-up 2 | PS–PS | 11.06 | 4.33 | −4.67 |
| (Three months) | PS–SR | 11.00 | 3.00 | −1.00 |
| | SR–SR | 1.16 | 1.90 | −0.80 |
| | SR–PS | 10.00 | 3.33 | −0.80 |
| | WLC–WLC | −1.16 | 0.00 | −0.05 |
| | WLC–IC | 2.20 | 2.30 | −1.67 |

[a] Negative values on the HAS indicate improvement.

[b] PS = Problem-solving training; SR = Social reinforcement for activity; WLC = Waiting-list control; IC = Information control

only the PS–PS and PS–SR groups maintained reductions on the Beck over the WLC–WLC group while, on the SRS, the PS–PS group maintained reduction over the WLC–WLC and continuous social reinforcement groups (SR–SR). Apparently, a problem-solving component is important in the reduction of depression in this population.

The combination of operant and cognitive methods to increase activity level has also been shown to be effective for reducing depression (Hussian, 1979). Alternating treatment designs were employed

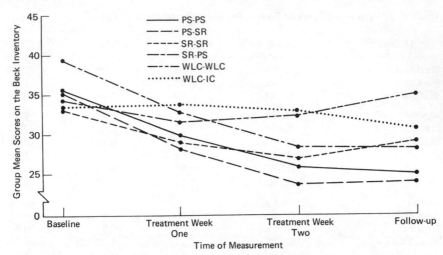

Figure 8-6.   Group Mean Scores on the Beck Depression Inventory.

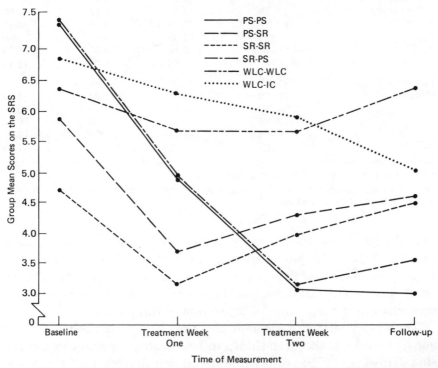

Figure 8-7.   Group Mean Scores on the Self-Rating Scale.

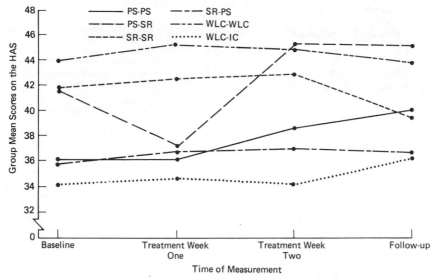

**Figure 8-8.   Group Mean Scores on the Hospital Adjustment Scale.**

to allow for a clear test of the relative superiority of the two approaches. Two residents were treated for depression while a third was treated for her high frequency verbalizations regarding dying. All three subjects were residents of a nursing home and were over sixty years of age.

The results from one subject are pictured in Figure 8-9. For this resident, selective reinforcement for participation in craft classes alone was randomly alternated with reinforcement plus positive coping statements such as "This place is home now and I'm going to make the most of it," or "If I feel a low spell coming on I'm going to fight it by keeping my mind active." The results show that the operant reinforcement therapy was enhanced by adding the cognitive component. The decrease in scores on the Beck Depression Inventory and a self-rating scale is more rapid when the coping statements are employed.

The results from the second resident showed the same enhancement with a decrease on the self-rating scale from 24 to 0. This reduction holds up even two months after treatment.

The third resident showed a marked reduction in the number of dying verbalizations through the use of an extinction procedure but

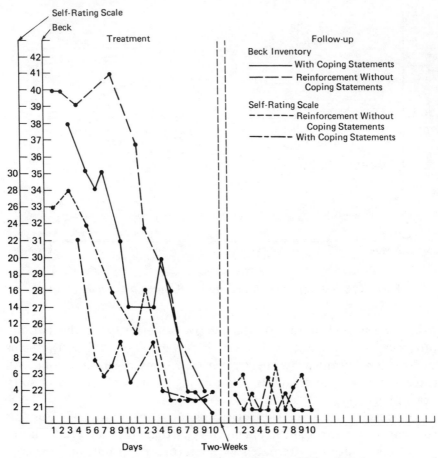

**Figure 8–9.  Therapeutic Program for Depression Combining Reinforcement and Coping Strategies.**

little maintenance at the two-week follow-up. At this point, a list of previously rehearsed self-instructions, such as "Just before I say that I'm dying I must think of three reasons for living," was handed to the subject before the experimenter turned away. Although little difference was evident through the treatment phase between the extinction alone and extinction plus self-instruction approaches, the enhanced maintenance phase indicates the additional benefit derived from the use of the combined procedure.

These findings suggest that the inclusion of cognitive treatment in the form of self-instructions or coping statements is effective and may facilitate the therapeutic process with geriatric patients. The results from the third subject may also suggest an increase in maintenance with the added cognitive component.

Depression has also been effectively reduced in geriatric patients through milieu therapy (Vickers, 1976) which combines drug, group, and attitude restructuring therapies; providing the elderly patient with more personal responsibility (Rodin & Langer, 1977); and short-term individualized psychotherapy (Willner, 1978). The mere reduction of the isolation factor has also been suggested as a possible therapeutic approach to reduce depression—as well as those behaviors which typically have been associated with "chronic brain syndrome" (Ernst, Badash, Beran, Kosovsky, & Kleinhauz, 1977; Ernst, Beran, Badash, Kosovsky, & Kleinhauz, 1977). Ernst, Beran, Safford, and Kleinhauz (1978, p. 473) make the following suggestions.

Thus, we conclude by stating that we believe that the therapist must not focus only on the organic factors of the aging brain but must stress the effects of the environment. He should conceptualize the relationship of organic and functional factors together with the development of mental disorders in the elderly as a cyclical process in order to find new tools for the treatment of his elderly patients. What has all too often been called chronic brain syndrome may be viewed as a complex of symptoms found among elderly persons who have, because of a combination of internal and external changes in their life, become isolated. Alleviation of this isolation may permit the therapist to treat those patients formerly called untreatable, and offers exciting leads toward the provision of preventative therapies to forestall future disorders in presently healthy, but aging, persons.

It is clear that such considerations require far-reaching design changes in current living facilities for the aged though the individual therapist may make relocation suggestions for his or her clients when isolation or stimulation deficits are present.

## Anxiety

One study by Garrison (1978) showed the successful application of stress management training with geriatric anxiety. The author's approach involved teaching the client to understand the nature of anxiety, muscular relaxation training, systematic desensitization, and meditation. The elderly patients completed the following procedure: Tension-relaxation alternation, relaxation alone, meditation while relaxed, differential and rapid relaxation, imagining the anxiety producing scene while relaxed, and a follow-up. Training lasted seven sessions, included homework and a two-month follow-up. The sessions were conducted in groups. The success of this procedure should encourage therapists to use standard behavioral techniques with this population.

This author utilized systematic desensitization with an eighty-three-year-old woman who reported feeling anxious when she was near persons exhibiting strange behavior or who were known to be "crazy." She was a resident in a facility in which many of the other residents had predominately psychiatric diagnoses and long histories of institutionalization for behavioral problems.

The rationale of systematic desensitization was given and the client and therapist formulated rational self-statements as responses incompatible with anxiety. Formal relaxation was not taught since the client was confined to a wheelchair and was also unable to tense her muscles adequately.

Table 8–3 shows the self-statements used in the two training sessions. Table 8–4 gives the twelve-step hierarchy developed by the client and therapist and the anxiety rating for each step. After five desensitization training sessions, one hour each session, the client could both imaginally, and *in vivo*, sit in the commons areas with low (no higher than 20 SUDs) level anxiety. The results were maintained at a three-week and six-month follow-up. By learning rational coping statements in addition to self-reinforcing nonavoidance behavior, this resident could now interact with the patients she chose without experiencing anticipatory anxiety. This case illustrates the use of response modification when the changing of environmental variables, in this case through relocation of the client or sedation of the other residents, is not possible.

Table 8-3  Rational Coping Statements Used in the Modification of Anxiety Concerning Proximity to Psychiatric Patients

1. Most of these people haven't shown any signs of cursing, fighting, or acting "different" in many years. They just need a place to stay like I do.
2. These people are controlled well on medication.
3. If a fight breaks out there are many staff members here to keep the other patients from getting involved.
4. On those few occasions when a problem occurs, the staff arrive so quickly that no one ever gets hurt.
5. I will not allow my fears to prevent me from enjoying the activities here.
6. If my fear begins to get overwhelming, I'll stop, take a few deep breaths, and think about my family coming next week.
7. I can always move out of the way if a problem arises.
8. There are many real nice people here to talk to. I'll not stay in my room all day and lose their contact and friendship.
9. I've learned to identify those changes in behavior which sometimes suggest a problem about to occur so I can move away.

Anxiety involving discrete stimuli was also effectively reduced by this author through the use of stress inoculation training. Four geriatric residents of a long-term care facility (mean age = 79) experienced extreme anxiety when imagining a ride on an elevator. None of these residents had ever been on an elevator in their lives and, prior to a facility-wide relocation, had had no need to have *in vivo* encounters with elevators. The move demanded that they use the elevators either for convenience or necessity (two residents were confined to wheelchairs). These residents had resigned themselves to remaining on the floors of their residence and had given up participating in outdoor activities. It became clear that *in vivo* exposure, no matter how gradual, would not meet with success so the stress inoculation procedure was described to these residents.

Informal relaxation, mostly covert, was utilized. The residents were told of the relationship between covert self-verbalizations and approach-avoidance behavior and anxiety. They were then instructed to tell the therapist, in a group, all the negative and "outlandish" things they thought about in connection with elevators. These verbalizations included feelings of entrapment, being buried alive, doors not reopening, being caught in the doors, and plummeting four sto-

Table 8-4   Hierarchy Used in the Systematic Desensitization of Anxiety Involving Psychiatric Patients

| SUDS rating | Hierarchy Item |
|---|---|
| 10 | Hearing a patient yelling down the hallway, talking in a confused manner. |
| 20 | Seeing a psychiatric patient passing in the hallway, hesitate outside your room, and move on. |
| 25 | Entering the commons area and seeing a psychiatric patient talking loudly or moving in an odd manner. |
| 30 | Sitting in the commons area and seeing two psychiatric patients staring at each other. |
| 40 | Sitting in the commons area seeing two or more psychiatric patients yelling at each other. |
| 45 | Sitting in the commons area seeing a group of two or more psychiatric patients moving toward you but still twenty or more feet away. |
| 50 | Sitting in the commons area and being approached by a psychiatric patient for a light or money. |
| 60 | Witnessing a verbal battle between two psychiatric patients twenty or more feet away. |
| 70 | Witnessing a verbal battle between two psychiatric patients right in front of your wheelchair. |
| 80 | Witnessing threatening posture between two psychiatric patients at a distance with nursing staff nearby. |
| 90 | Witnessing the beginnings of a scuffle with nursing staff nearby. |
| 100 | You're the only one in the area of a fight between two psychiatric patients several feet away and your wheelchair is backed in a corner. |

ries into the ground. After informal relaxation, an educational phase was conducted in which diagrams of elevators, safety measures, inspection license, and general operation was discussed. As can be seen in Figures 8-10 and 8-11, little approach behavior resulted during this phase.

In the third phase, positive verbalizations were constructed, and the residents practiced these statements aloud and covertly for three days in half-hour sessions. These statements included, "When the doors open, I am confidently going inside and hold onto the rail" and "If the doors stick I will not panic but will press the red button until help arrives."

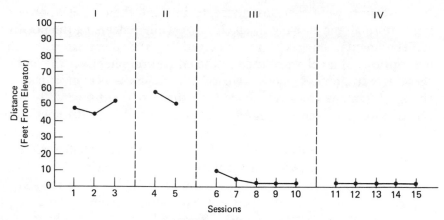

Figure 8-10.

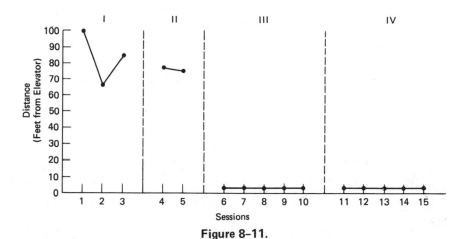

Figure 8-11.

Figures 8-10—8-12. Randomly Chosen Patients' Progress through Stress Inoculation Training to Reduce Anxiety Concerning Elevators.

Figure 8-10 represents Patient #2, Figure 8-11 represents Patient #3. Phase I = Baseline; Phase II = Education phase; Phase III = Stress-inoculation; Phase IV = Two-month follow-up.

The clients were then instructed to imagine themselves approaching, entering, and moving in an elevator while rehearsing the positive self-statements. Images were enhanced by the therapist using the descriptions of an elevator used in the education phase. At the end of these five training sessions, two of the residents accompanied the therapist in a one-story ride while the other two went separately with the therapist. As can be seen in Figures 8–10 and 8–11 distance from the elevators was decreased until the residents could ride on the elevators with anxiety ratings of two or below on a ten-point scale (see Figure 8–12). On a two-month follow-up, all four residents were riding on the elevators with minimal anxiety several times a day. They expressed satisfaction with their self-rated anxiety levels as well.

Less situation specific anxiety has also been successfully treated through stress-inoculation training. Through the use of more generalized statements which could be applied to any routinely encountered situation, overall anxiety levels were reported by almost all clients as being satisfactory. Particularly useful is exaggeration of the anxiety-producing situation during the exposure phase. For example, an elderly client who has partial paralysis and is anxious about losing his or her independence and mobility may be asked to imagine themselves more totally disabled. Positive coping statements are then taught to constructively deal with this more debilitating circumstance. The exposure phase may also be effectively conducted by

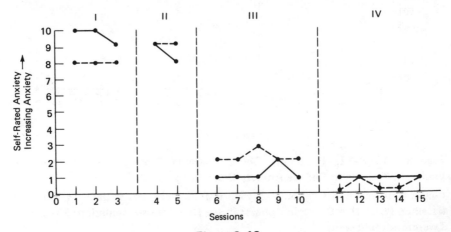

Figure 8–12.

actually limiting the client physically in correspondence to the excess disability in order to more accurately represent the fear-producing situation.

## Paranoid Thought

Concentration on the possibility of dire consequences or attracting someone's dislike disrupts on-going rational thought and constructive behavior. Two approaches with elements of behavioral technology have been applied successfully in this difficult problem area.

First, rational restructuring, whereby the client's irrational chain of cognitions is broken down by analysis and confrontation with rational alternatives, may be useful. Often, the chain of paranoid thoughts continue to snowball, maintained by the consequences of earlier expressions of irrationality such that the individual loses track of the inappropriateness of their ruminations and fear. The following case illustrates the restructuring process.

A sixty-seven-year-old female resident of a long-term care facility expressed thoughts of being killed by unknown assailants while she slept. For approximately two weeks she slept an average of two hours a night, consumed fewer than 1500 calories a day, and was in constant fear of her prediction. After these two weeks, the therapist began cognitive restructuring along with relaxation training. The patient was trained to substitute more rational statements for the previously rehearsed ones. Instead of concentrating on such thoughts as, "They tell me I'm going to be shot," and "A man told me he was going to kill me next Thursday," the patient was told to think, "I have thought I would be killed now for two weeks and not a thing has happened, I must be making these things up," or "I have never hurt anyone in my life, no one has a reason for wanting me killed." The client was asked to keep a diary of the paranoid thoughts as they occurred. After four weeks of relaxation and the rehearsal of positive counter-statements, the client's appetite returned to normal, she began sleeping an average of six hours, and she reported not hearing the voices again. She stated that she felt so stupid now but those voices were so very real at the time. She stated that the diary which she kept was the most important part of the approach since constant reminders that the appointed date of termination had repeatedly passed uneventfully finally extinguished the statements.

Another approach, one which is perhaps more likely in a geriatric facility given the frequent adherence to medical approaches, is the combination of the behavioral methodology above with a pharmacological approach.

A sixty-two-year-old woman verbalized thoughts of being targeted for poison for some dreadful act which she had supposedly committed when younger. She had withdrawn to her room, with the curtains drawn, for two months prior to referral to a psychologist. The behavior had gotten to the point where she was extremely weak and anemic as a result of the nonconsumption of food. The urgency of the problem suggested that a drug regimen would be most appropriate for a rapid return to levels which might permit a behavioral approach. Approximate food consumption, hours slept, and the number of paranoid thoughts served as criteria variables. Treatment with thiothixene was then begun. After four days the client's appetite improved slightly and her sleep returned to acceptable ranges (mean per night = 4.5 hours). However, around the fifth day following treatment the gains leveled off and the client continued to voice the suspicions regarding future harm. A cognitive restructuring and relaxation program was begun on day twelve. In this case, however, the client was asked, while relaxed, to imagine the fearful situation (i.e., hearing the threats, tasting a peculiar taste in her food, getting nauseous, etc.) and to counter the fear with the more rational, positive statements. The medication was continued through this stage. After six sessions, the client's appetite had returned to normal (approximately 3500 calories), sleep duration was 6.5 hours per night, and she no longer reported hearing the incessant voice. The medication was terminated about six weeks later and the client reports that the voice has not returned at a two-month follow-up.

Further research on the combination of pharmacological and behavioral approaches is needed, not just in the treatment of paranoia,

but all the problems in geriatric psychology. In addition, the pharmacology literature would be improved greatly by employing the designs
used by behavior therapists to verify treatment effects.

## Other Problem Areas and Techniques

Several other behavior modification techniques may be useful in the
reduction of incompatible responses in the elderly. The use of extinction procedures are extremely effective with geriatric clients.
Particularly, the use of "time-out" in cases of chronic complaints is
appropriate. Assertiveness training, specifically designed to train
those responses which are effective in situations involving loss of
self-determination, passivity brought about by relocation, and being
taken for granted by insensitive others, may also be effective. Inappropriate response to the conditions which society and the elderly
clients themselves impose may be replaced by more active responses
which meet with reinforcement from others or from the impact
that these new responses have on the environment. It is important
that, during therapy with elderly clients, the clinician is sensitive to
the response of appropriate assertiveness and does not extinguish
such responses or approximations of the response.

Modeling is also an effective behavioral approach either in the
building of response adequacy or in the vicarious learning of more
appropriate responses. The power of modeling effects is very noticeable in geriatric facilities in the building of inappropriate responses
and should be recognized as an etiological variable as well as a
therapeutic approach. For example, the author is familiar with two
instances of rapidly "spreading" pathological behavior which was
almost entirely instigated and maintained by modeling. An outbreak
of psychoneurodermatitis spread throughout five wings of a nursing
facility though there were only two or three true cases of scabies.
Skin breakdown, rashes, itching, and redness occurred in a majority
of the residents and quite a few of the staff members. A combination
of modeled responses, observations of differential attention, and
fear created an atmosphere of symptom preoccupation. In the other
case, four residents of one wing in another long-term care facility
began verbalizing paranoid thoughts. Individual therapy helped to
alleviate the problem by providing social reinforcement for non-

paranoid verbalizations and extinction of speech which contained references to being killed, harmed, or shipped to a mental institution. Although only one resident had exhibited a history of such behavior, these other three patients had shown the same set of behaviors.

These cases suggest that modeling may have an impact on the reduction of inappropriate responses as well. Observations of others engaged in activities, others being placed in a "time-out" room, and others overcoming fears regarding ambulation, help to eliminate similar responses in the observer. It would be valuable to determine the parameters of modeling as a treatment approach with elderly clients such as the characteristics of the model which differentially effect the learning of the modeled response.

## Reattribution

A frequently encountered problem in practice with elderly clients is misattribution. Often, a behavior or set of behaviors is perceived by the client as indicating some nonmodifiable or otherwise frightening clinical entity such as deterioration, disease, or tissue pathology. These observations and the subsequent labeling can then cause excessive ruminations, anxiety, withdrawal, and depression. It is often the case that a half an hour to an hour conference of an educational nature with the client is sufficient to eliminate the misattribution and, quite immediately, the undesirable behavioral response. Assigning causality to external events rather than more damaging internal attributes is the desired goal (Sparacino, 1978). If the imparting of information alone is not enough, introducing another elderly client who underwent the same debilitating attribution process but who is now functioning appropriately is almost always sufficient to reduce the inappropriate responding. The client can then inform interested family members and friends as to the true nature of the problem, thus resulting in less anxiety for all persons involved. Cases which were discussed in Chapter 4 involving medication-induced dystonia and the relationship between damage in the basal ganglia and crying behavior are examples of potential misattributional behavior. The following case describes the process of reattribution therapy in more detail.

A sixty five year-old resident of a long-term care facility was referred for rapid onset anxiety and nervousness. On interview, he appeared anxious, showed a short attention span, motor restlessness, and upper extremity tremors. The client was told of the nature of a new medication which he was taking (haliperidol), the frequency of these physical symptoms due to such medication, and the relationship between these tremors which he had observed and the attribution of physical deterioration which he had made. Then, the relationship between self-labeling and anxiety was discussed. Prior to the prescribing of an anti-Parkinson drug, the client stated that he felt better and he returned to his prior level of activity engagement. The tremors, though still present in a less intense form, no longer distracted this man from participating in favored activities.

Though a reattributional approach usually is successful in the elimination of such inappropriate labeling, prevention of the original misattribution would be more desirable than intervention at a later date. Prophylaxis would involve little more than having the physician or physician's representative describe the side-effects which may be expected to occur as a result of the consumption of a given medication or an interaction. Sensitivity on the part of all professionals dealing with elderly clients may also prevent misattribution involving other physical symptoms such as the development of cataracts, transient ischemic attacks, and age-related memory decline. The prospect of irreversible visual impairment, permanent unsteadiness or loss of feeling, or senility due to these processes could understandably lead to self-defeating responses.

Reattribution as a therapeutic approach fits nicely into the compensatory model. For instance, the number of times that statements such as, "Well Doc, I guess I'm getting senile," or "It was just a matter of time. Both my parents got like this before they died," are encountered in practice with elderly clients is enormous. The most frightening aspect of this frequently encountered set of self-verbalizations is that they may lead to further self-deprecation, isolation, and passive acceptance on the part of the client and others. When this is allowed to continue, negative consequences may result.

It is a simple matter, however, to refocus the elderly client's attention on more important concerns and more accurate information and away from the erroneous assignment of causality.

## MODIFICATION OF STIMULI

The final area of psychotherapeutic intervention involves changing impinging stimuli in order to effect a change in response. Therapeutic approaches which are primarily concerned with the stimulus variables include milieu therapy, total systems design, and shaping and fading procedures (Mishara, 1978; Pfeiffer, 1972). Usually, these approaches are, as described in Chapters 3 and 7, used with more severe geriatric problems. However, two areas which involve primarily considerations at the input level, total systems design and relocation effects, may involve all elderly persons regardless of their mental status.

### System-wide Changes

Brezinski, Jones, Atkinson, and Noah (1977) have shown, with a sample of 195 institutionalized residents, the powerful effects of environmental design features on the maintenance of skills. Using a time-sampling procedure, these authors found slight to moderate improvements in mobility, verbal interaction, self-care, and activity due to specially designed living systems. The design of total living environments is probably the best way of insuring continuity of controlling factors. The main drawback of such an approach is that new structures must be built which increase the likelihood that group interactions, continence, safe ambulation, self-feeding, recreation, self-medication and other desirable behaviors are likely to result. Behavioral engineering of total systems may be accomplished in part now by educating those who deliver health care within existing geriatric facilities as to behavioral principles. The application of timely and consistent reinforcement, the turning away from undesirable but nondangerous behavior, and the awareness of learning principles and compensatory behavior are desirable goals of this educational process. A sample in-service program is presented in the next chapter.

While prophylactic environmental aides such as those described by

Cautela (1972) and total systems planning are the end-products of long-term and insightful planning, we are still faced with the problem of controlling stimulus events in existing environments in order to balance those factors which contribute to efficient medical service delivery and those which involve independence, stimulation, interactions, activity, and self-directed behavior. Unfortunately, the contingencies which are regulated by governmental agencies are not yet those which "encourage" new design ideas or implementation. Anyone who has witnessed a review panel's on-site activity in a nursing home or is acquainted with the elements with which this panel is most concerned quickly realizes that the quality of psychological care which the elderly receive in most geriatric facilities is not the primary target for improvement.

## Relocation

The effects of relocation of elderly individuals to new residences are well documented (e.g., Killian, 1970; Lawton & Yaffe, 1970; Pino, Rosica, & Carter, 1978). These effects have included increased mortality and morbidity rates beyond those expected. From the literature, though, several possible techniques may be used which have resulted oftentimes, in no increases in either area.

1. Brezinski, Jones, Atkinson, and Noah (1977) gradually adapted residents to their new living quarters. This gradual exposure prior to the move is thought to reduce premove anticipatory anxiety and the stress associated with unfamiliar quarters. Prior site visitation should also minimize the typical effects of relocation.

2. It is often impractical to utilize site visitation when the resident to be relocated is physically unable to tolerate travel beyond that required for the move. However, pictures or films of the new facility and reports from other residents may substitute quite adequately for *in vivo* exposure. Information and constructive guides may accompany the visual presentation such that the presentation takes the form of prophylactic stress-inoculation or desensitization training.

3. The effects of modeling, guided participation, and the presence of a confidante may be combined in a "buddy system" approach to relocation. If an entire facility is to be relocated, the staff could pair-off elderly individuals who would visit the site together before the

move and move together. Particularly good models may be used for several problem residents.

4. Special attention should be placed on identification of high-frequency routes or services within the new facility and special markers used to identify these routes and service functions. Features which are present in the new facility which were not present in the prior facility or are radically different should be marked clearly using large colored stimuli.

5. Familiar objects and personal items should precede the relocated residents and be in place when the residents arrive. A favorite chair, picture, or bedspread increases the continuity between sites.

Close observation should be made of elderly individuals after changes in residence. Problems with adjustment should be addressed quickly before they lead to pathological response. Drastic increases over base rate mortality or morbidity at postrelocation are preventable so it is essential to exercise diligence during this time.

## THERAPIST VARIABLES

The treatment techniques described in this chapter differ little from standard applications in the general population. The fact that there are data, though far from substantial, to support the application of such techniques will, hopefully, encourage their utilization. Admittedly, there are problems which are associated with this population for which the behavior therapist is not particularly well prepared or where the supportive literature is nonexistent. However, even in the areas which are not well represented such as terminal illness, grief, and dying, adjunctive behaviors (which contribute greatly to a successful practice) coupled with the sound application of presently known behavioral techniques should be most efficient in dealing with even these unexplored problems. Though one would be hard pressed to argue that success in therapy is simply a matter of the positive characteristics of the therapist (i.e., warmth, empathy, honesty, sensitivity, acceptance, unconditional positive regard) and, in fact, success may be achieved in the absence of such variables, there is no doubt that a clinician with a large number of certain clients (e.g., terminally ill or grieving) relies on these ambiguous qualities quite often. For it is when the therapist must sit quietly and listen that these responses, or the lack thereof, are most obvious.

A significant part of the geriatric psychologist's time is involved in dealing with an elderly client's (and his or her family's) response to dying or significant loss. It is most important in such cases to employ a variety of approaches in order to control pain, reduce anxiety, train constructive approaches to deal with planning, and to replace misinformation regarding the course of the illness. However, it is critical for the therapist to remember that he or she is a stimulus-generator and, while in the presence of the client, these stimuli affect the client's response even when these stimuli are not a part of a therapeutic regimen. One should use these nonspecific characteristics judiciously.

# 9
# Behavior Therapy in Long-Term Care Facilities

Although the geriatric population exhibits more psychological problems than any other generation, it is a fact that deliverers of psychological services seldom come in contact with this high-risk group. There is, however, certainly no deficiency in the numbers of service providers. The problem to overcome, then, is either access, willingness, or both. We can do little more to encourage willingness, at least on the part of the practitioner, so the discussion will be limited to access. It will be argued that one setting in which access should present little problem is in the nursing home, and yet there are very few psychologists who have a majority of their practice in this setting. Several points of support for the presence of a psychologist in nursing homes or at least in consultation with nursing home personnel are available. Representative duties, responsibilities, and referral practices will also be discussed.

## CLINICAL PSYCHOLOGY IN THE NURSING HOME

A special subcommittee of the United States Senate (1974) reported that in that year there were over 950,000 elderly persons in nursing homes in this country. In 1972, for the first time in history, Medicaid paid out more for nursing home care than for care provided at general hospitals. The fact that there are approximately 22 million Americans who are at least age sixty-five and not presently in nursing homes should not dilute one's interest in what continues to be a very significant number of people.

Second, most of the truly bothersome, severe, and progressively deteriorating behavior problems of the elderly are represented in nursing-home residents. Due to the high frequency of physical problems, the number of drug prescriptions, positively skewed economic distribution, decentralization philosophy of regional mental institutions, and the attributes of some of these facilities themselves, these severe problems are statistically overrepresented. Also, long-term care facilities typically house patients who are neither elderly nor physically limited. It is not uncommon to find a wide variety of ages and psychiatric diagnoses on the censuses of most long-term care facilities. This is particularly true in those facilities which include beds not designated for skilled care. We should be interested, of course, in offering services where they are most needed.

Third, skilled nursing, retirement, respite, and intermediate-care facilities of any size are potentially ideal environments in which to effect behavior change. For behaviorally oriented clinicians particularly (but not exclusively) the usual problems of uncontrollable extrinsic life-changes and noncompliance with homework or rehearsal are less problematic. The presence of a "captive audience," capability for around-the-clock observation, and potential modeling effects, also promote more efficient behavior change programs than found in traditional settings such as outpatient clinics, mental health centers, or in private practice.

Fourth, as Hyerstoy (1979) points out, the peculiar skills and knowledge which a psychologist can offer are well-suited for a variety of purposes in long-term care facilities. She describes a variety of roles which a psychologist can fill or contribute to such as serving as a patient advocate, diagnostician (assessor), therapist, researcher, liaison with community agencies, a modifier of attitudes with regard to aging, consultant, and as a program developer. More specifically, an individual with a degree in psychology may effectively contribute to such nondirect patient care areas as personnel selection and promotion, public relations, dietary service systems, communication skills, management skills, staff report writing, in-service training, and family services.

The potential areas for input by psychologists in long-term care are vast. Much of this input could probably be delivered independent of the training and orientation of the psychologist. However, there are several important reasons why a psychologist trained in the experimental/clinical model, which is the basis for behavioral training, promotes human service delivery in such facilities more adequately than is possible with clinicians exposed to any other background.

## THE BEHAVIOR THERAPIST IN LONG-TERM CARE

A psychologist who is trained with an emphasis on the behavioral model enhances geriatric care for a variety of reasons. Concern with the training of mediators, the collection of data, the administration of criteria measures, and continuity of application, maintenance, and generalization, parallels the concerns of long-term care. Operating within a functional analysis approach, regardless of the problem area, will meet with a high probability of success. The behavior thera-pist's efforts to operationally define problems, delineate specific subgoals and tactics, and empirically validate his or her methods not only results in greater accountability and a reduction in wasted time, but also results in patient care planning which can be more easily carried out by paraprofessionals. The delivery of this care may also more easily be evaluated by outside peer reviews and third-party reimbursers.

The fact that behavioral approaches tend to involve methods which are easily identifiable and which entail specifically described target behaviors increases the public nature of the therapeutic activity. This in turn provides interested observers with the type of information regarding that activity which lends itself to ethical scrutiny. Several authors (Berkowitz, 1978; MacDonald, 1976) have addressed these considerations in long-term care and similar facilities. The utilization of scientific recording methods and data collection in general encourages review for accountability. In nursing facilities this exposure potential is highly desirable since the client population consists of a significant proportion of individuals who cannot give informed consent or disengage from participation once the intervention has started. An established record of success and the high visibility of behavioral intervention are persuasive arguments for adopting such methodology in these settings.

Staff training, a forum for the consideration of ethical questions, the referral system, and professional cooperation remain to be discussed.

## IN-SERVICE TRAINING

The sine qua non of an effective behavioral program in any facility is knowledgeable and consistent application of behavioral methodology by everyone who has significant contact with the clients being served. The clinician cannot rely on word-of-mouth communication or other less formal means of education because of high staff turnover rates, multiple shifts, and lack of previous contact with behavioral methodology, characteristics of many inpatient settings. Therefore, a well-designed in-service which is offered regularly, geared toward several levels of comprehension, and accompanied by periodic prompts and careful monitoring is necessary. Since it is economically unfeasible and probably not desirable to completely isolate high-risk patients, the entire health-care staff, especially the entire nursing service hierarchy, needs to be included in formal classroom or workshop activities.

The possible content of the classroom presentation of behavioral principles includes the following content areas. Acquired skill or knowledge in these areas has proven to be effective in maintaining quality psychological care when accompanied by more intense individual intervention by the clinician.

1. An introduction to the behavioral approach should include its basis in laboratory and controlled research. Discussions of the myths surrounding "behaviorism" (e.g., behaviorism is equivalent to psychosurgery, the implantation of electrodes, shock treatment, drug therapy, and other "will-destroying" atrocities) are also essential before proceeding to other matters.

2. An explanation of the benefits of a scientific psychology, in-

cluding the concepts of prediction and control and the undesirability of making inferences from observable behavior to underlying hypothetical constructs.

3. A description of the S–O–R–C model with examples of the sub-variables and the application of functional analysis should be presented early in the course.

4. The basic principles of reinforcement, punishment, and extinction should be simply introduced. The common-sense appeal of a statement such as, "If you want a behavior to increase in frequency, follow it with something positive and if you want a behavior to decrease in frequency, follow it with something aversive or at least not positive," is perhaps more important for teaching purposes than the amendments and qualifications which more sophisticated exploration reveals. Examples of positive reinforcers and the concepts of consistency, contingency, and immediacy should also be routinely included.

5. The concept and procedural aspects of extinction should be described in some depth. Punishment in such a setting tends to be associated with conditioned responses which may prevent acceptance and is not an important procedure for paraprofessional mediators to master. Particular attention should be paid to the illustration of the phenomenon of transient behavioral increases immediately following the initiation of an extinction or "time-out" program. Many of the nursing personnel and other staff members have shown a low threshold for behavioral excesses and they need to be informed of this artifact before they experience it. It is more beneficial for the nonprofessional staff to predict the outcome of intervention, even when the outcome is less than desirable, than for them to have early doubts about the efficacy of one component of the training.

6. A brief acquaintance with behavioral indices to be monitored follows. Teaching observational skills includes attention to potentially meaningful changes in patients' behavior such as a neglect of personal appearance, restlessness, withdrawal, self-deprecatory statements, crying spells, loss of appetite, and changes in sleep patterns. Also included are common drug-induced negative side-effects presented in nontechnical language, such as tremors, shuffling gait, complaints of urinary retention, repetitive muscle movements, fixed gaze, fly-catcher movements of the tongue, and other commonly

observed responses to pharmacological agents in the elderly population. Particularly effective, either with an entire class or later in smaller groups, is a "grand round" format which includes presentation of drug-induced behaviors which are awaiting modification or are, regrettably, irreversible.

7. A variety of behavioral programs should be discussed with particular attention to the roles that the variety of staff members play in these programs. The urinary incontinence program is a good starting place since the procedures are relatively simple and the theoretical nature of temporal conditioning, feedback, and reinforcement is simply and interestingly presentable. Also, success with this program is highly probable, thus resulting in fairly reliable, prompt reinforcement for its application by the trainees.

Empirically validated behavioral programs which may be presented at either level of training may also include procedures for eliminating wandering, individual therapy programs aimed at a variety of response classes, instructions for maintaining 24-hour reality orientation programing, suicide precautions and observation procedures, and symptoms of drug-induced side effects in problem patients.

8. Some form of performance evaluation should be conducted before and immediately following the classroom activities, including pre- and post-test controls for the varied levels of background sophistication while permitting assessment of the training package. A sample in-service, multiple-choice test is presented in Appendix B.

Beyond this introductory content material, more advanced classes can be presented as needed to the appropriate staff members (e.g., LPN's and RN's). These classes may include a sample from the areas of stimulus control, cognitive restructuring techniques, the inadequacy of psychodiagnostic labels, and neuropsychological signs. Particularly astute individuals may even be designated to receive special training in behavioral observation methodology, calculations of reliability, and other data collection techniques which would not interfere greatly with their daily routine.

The purposes of such training are two-fold, then. An introductory and terminal exposure is offered to a majority of the staff for purposes of being able to observe for changes as well as to insure that, at the very least, they do not interfere with ongoing behavioral programs. Secondly, a select sample of that audience may be chosen for more intense training so as to become more active behavior-therapy mediators (Lee, 1969).

The procedural aspects of the training, such as class size, class length, type of interactions and presentation, the types of personnel to invite (or require) attendance, the number of classes, and the type of follow-up or evaluation will generally be dictated by the needs of the client population, the size of the facility, and the cooperation of the administrative staff. One effective method currently employed at one long-term care facility in North Carolina with which the author was affiliated, includes a brief introduction to all new employees during the mandatory orientation period, a routine hour-long class approximately every six months, random spot checks of charting and activity on a daily basis, and periodic memos on pertinent procedures or weak-spots as needed. All nursing personnel from the aide level to the Director of Nursing, and all other employees with patient contact are included in the above educational process. The hour-long formal presentations are offered at times conducive for the inclusion of nursing personnel from all three shifts, though more concentrated efforts are directed at the two daytime shifts.

As might be surmised, staff cooperation and continued attention to behavioral concerns is maintained only when such cooperation and attention results in contingent positive consequences. Behavioral in-services may be worked into a pre-existing training program (with its own contingencies) or special considerations may be employed. These considerations may include recognizing such behavior in the promotion or merit system, special recognition awards at monthly or yearly intervals, small cash bonuses delivered on a random basis or variable interval schedule, or recognition on a similar schedule in facility newsletters or special memos. Compliance in this regard will be less than adequate without such contingencies since newly acquired skills are being required which are not necessarily self-maintaining.

## ETHICAL PROTECTIONS

Two factors with regard to behavioral intervention in long-term care facilities tend to result in the generation of ethical considerations above and beyond the usual questions of decency, positive regard, and legality. These factors are the nature of the population and the nature of behavior therapy itself.

Responsibility for decisions concerning rights to determine the disposition of one's own body and the extensions thereof are relatively clear cut in children, unimpaired adults, and individuals who have been declared incompetent by judicial process. Persons residing in institutions who are not there by choice also have extrinsic sources of concern and advocacy. This is not usually true when the subject is an elderly person residing in a long-term care facility. Oftentimes the individual is impaired to such an extent that a unanimous decision regarding the level of competence can be made. However, there may be no responsible party and, in fact, there may be no party interested at all in the disposition of the elderly client. Nor is it probable that a formal proceeding to judge the level of competency has been conducted so no responsible party has been assigned. In confronting these frequent realities the therapist finds him or herself in an uncomfortable bind. Unlike the medical practitioner, it is not quite so easy to argue that intervention is to alleviate a life-threatening condition so, in order to prevent aversive events from occurring to the clinician, no intervention of any kind is attempted. This passive behavior could then be construed as a violation of that patient's rights, or the rights of other patients in the vicinity.

In the case of research and the use of innovative or aversive treatment strategies the potential for abuse and, on the other side of the coin, neglect, exist. Even when the patient appears, by unanimous consent, to be capable of understanding procedures and giving informed consent, some have argued that the very nature of the institution, that of health-care provider, dilutes the act of consent. Even when alternative intervention techniques are explained, the dangers of the proposed technique provided, or the voluntariness of the participation stressed, the dependent nature of the patient in the patient-provider relationship is thought to taint the motivation to participate.

There are no expedient answers to these dilemmas, nor should there be. However, the behavioral clinician and/or researcher may find both legal and ethical relief from an institutional review board. Whether based upon the concept of diffusion of responsibility or the effectiveness of multiple, objective perceptions, these in-house review boards are extremely valuable to the consumer, the practitioner, the facility, and the community as a whole. Progress in areas that have little or no acceptable data base depends upon the assumption of risks which need to be regulated and monitored by a third party. The appearance of legislated protection devices such as patients' Bill of Rights have made such a practice a necessity. Again, drawing on the enlightened approach of one long-term care facility, the procedures in setting up such a review board are described.

## Authorization

The administration, in the interest of encouraging research in the area of long-term care, making available innovative treatment techniques, and promoting and protecting the rights of the patient, directed the formation of an in-house Ethics Committee with the following directives, objectives, and membership:

## Directives and Objectives

1. To review research proposals submitted to the committee by the administrator or a duly appointed representative (in his/her absence) for the purpose of protecting the rights and dignity of the patient during and following the course of any research project.

2. To review treatment proposals submitted to the committee by the administrator or a duly appointed representative (in his/her absence) for the purpose of protecting the rights and dignity of the patient during and following the course of the proposed treatment procedure. The proposal being submitted to the administrator may come from the therapist him/herself or from any other staff member concerned about the ethical implications of such a procedure.

**Membership.** Membership on the Ethics Committee is composed of roughly, half staff members and half nonstaff members. The original members of the Ethics Committee included outside members for the following reasons.

1. To enhance objectivity in the decision-making process by including outside members who offer a noninstitutional perspective.

2. To include a variety of expertise, some of which cannot be obtained from in-house staff members.

3. To insure that decisions would be made independently of the employer-employee relationship. To minimize this potential for

conflict-of-interest outside members were chosen who are not to be paid by the facility.

Other individuals may, at times, be present at the meetings as invited by the Ethics Committee or the administrator but they will not enjoy voting privileges.

## Process

The Ethics Committee serves in an advisory capacity to the administrator. The administrator has the final decision as to the implementation of the research project or treatment program.

The internal procedures, format, and activities of the Ethics Committee are determined by a majority vote of the members of the Ethics Committee subject to the approval of the administrator.

## Format for Proposal Review

1. A copy of the proposal is given to the administrator for his/her determination of implementation within the facility. At the discretion of the administrator ten (10) copies of the proposal are submitted by the proposee to the Ethics Committee.

2. The proposal is reviewed by a quorum of the Ethics Committee. A *quorum* has been determined to be "at least three staff members and three nonstaff members." The review is to be conducted in a group format and no proposal will be voted upon without a review before a quorum of Ethics Committee members.

3. If all members of the quorum of Ethics Committee members vote to endorse the proposal the project is considered as endorsed by all members of the Ethics Committee. *Endorsement* has been determined to be "unanimous approval of those voting."

4. Following the endorsement the proposee and the administrator are notified of the decision and the review is complete. Notification of endorsement is in the form of a recommendation to the administrator and the decision to implement the project is subject to his/her final approval.

5. If the proposal fails to be approved unanimously (endorsed) by the voting members (quorum) the proposee is notified. The proposee may then take appropriate action to rectify the objections

and then to resubmit the modified proposal to the quorum for review as above. If the proposee does not take action to rectify the objections the proposee may then resubmit the proposal as is to the quorum for review and discussion. The issue is then to be resolved and the proposee and the administrator are notified of the action taken by the Ethics Committee. In the case of nonunanimous voting on the resubmitted proposal, the administrator is provided with the results of the voting, a summary of the consenting opinion and a summary of the dissenting opinion. The administrator will make the final decision as to the implementation of the project within the facility whether the proposal receives endorsement (unanimous approval) or fails to receive endorsement (nonunanimous voting).

**Structure of the Proposal.** The Ethics Committee has adopted for use with all research proposals the following format, each item of which must be addressed by the investigator before the proposal will be considered for discussion.

1. What is the nature of your sample? (This brief description should include age, health status, sex, and other pertinent subject characteristics.)

2. In what setting will the study be conducted? (Lounge, patient rooms, etc.)

3. Will your subjects provide informed consent before participating?

4. Are participants informed about the nature of the experiment before it begins? (This item deals with the use of deception in the experimental design. If the response is "No," a rationale must accompany the proposal.)

5. Are participants explicitly given the option to withdraw from the experiment? (This must be answered in the affirmative and acts only as a cue to the investigator.)

6. Will the physician's approval be sought for each subject's participation? If not, why? (The physician and the potential subject should decide if the subject is capable of enduring the task. The Ethics Committee will make a recommendation as to whether or not this must be answered in the affirmative for each proposal.)

7. Will the administrator be given a list of proposed subjects? If not, why? (The administrator should decide, with consultation from

appropriate staff members, whether he/she feels that the potential subject is capable of entering into an informed consent agreement. In some cases, the Ethics Committee may recommend that this process be waived in the interest of confidentiality or the integrity of the experimental design.)

8. Are aversive stimuli being used and what are the steps taken to protect the participant from physical discomfort, harm, or mental stress? Explain. (An affirmative response acts as a cue for further exploration by the Ethics Committee.)

9. Does your study involve deception? (An affirmative response dictates that a rationale for the use of deception be included with the proposal.)

10. Will information obtained from a participant be kept confidential? If not, explain.

11. If information will not be kept confidential, will the participant be informed that others may have access to the information? (Whenever individuals other than the named researchers and the participant have access to such information, a statement of this nature must be placed in the consent form.)

12. Statement of purpose.

13. The experimental method. (State clearly the independent and dependent variables. Include any information concerning ethical considerations that you may have about this study and how you intend to deal with those concerns.) This description should be stated in nontechnical terms for the benefit of the members of the Ethics Committee.

14. If appropriate, will you offer treatment to the no-treatment or waiting-list control group(s)? (This item must be answered in the affirmative and carried out by the investigator(s) or other designated and appropriate parties for all proposals involving treatment outcome studies.)

15. Has the proposal been submitted to or accepted by another agency's Ethics Committee?

16. State the significance of your research for this facility, the participants, the elderly, or for science in general.

17. Experimenter(s)' qualifications. (This should include past experience in research, credentials, affiliations, etc., for each person involved in the research project.)

18. Do you agree to provide the facility with a copy of the results and/or publication reprint? (This item must be answered in the affirmative and acts only as a cue to the investigator.)

19. Subject consent form attached? (This item must be answered in the affirmative with the necessary attachment(s) and acts only as a cue to the investigator.)

20. Subject debriefing form attached? If no, explain. (A written debriefing form must be attached to the proposal unless the Ethics Committee waives this requirement for a particular proposal.)

21. The following statement should be included with signatures of the investigators below:

"I certify that every experimenter who is engaged in this research has been thoroughly trained in the procedures and methods to be used. I further acknowledge that every such experimenter has been thoroughly exposed to and briefed on the APA ethics concerning the use of human subjects in psychological research. I accept full responsibility for the ethical conduct of all persons assisting in this research." (Copies of these ethical principles will be made available to the investigator(s).)

**Structure of the Proposal (Innovative Treatment).** Proposals for the implementation of behavioral, or other, treatment techniques where existing empirical validation is minimal also include considerations of consent, information provided prior to release of consent, physician's approval, protective measures, confidentiality, and purpose. An acceptable proposal would also include data which demonstrates the clinician's awareness of alternative methods, the relative risks of the proposed treatment and of these alternatives, probability of success, history of outcome with more traditional techniques or an explanation of factors which prohibit the use of standard techniques, proposed duration of treatment, and the criteria employed to monitor and determine success of the approach.

The intent suggested by these procedures is perhaps more important than the procedures themselves. Essentially, the rights of the client to self-determination must be recognized and protected. A balance between the rights to treatment and research participation and the right to be free from trivial and possibly damaging manipulation must be achieved. It is not sufficient, however, to simply acknowledge the stickiness of the situation. Constructive, aggressive efforts must be instigated and maintained in those situations in which the slightest doubt exists with regard to the ethicality of a procedure. Administrators of long-term care facilities and other homes for the aged need to be cognizant of these concerns and professionals who provide care or conduct research in such facilities must be directed by them.

## PERTINENT ISSUES IN LONG-TERM CARE

The nature of long-term care is correlated with other issues which need to be addressed. The issues presented here are, of course, not exhaustive but should include some of the more relevant and facility-specific problem areas.

### Preoccupation with Management Problems

An issue that is constantly raised in nursing facilities by virtue of the characteristics of clients and the deficits in the training of the staff is behavior management. Despite in-service training emphasizing other issues, a preponderance of this author's referrals in a long-term care facility were, initially, patients who were creating a disturbance of the ongoing activities in the facility. Of course, these behaviors may well be ones which are creating problems for the person exhibiting the disturbances (as may be the case with loud crying episodes, multiple complaints, and insomnia), but the conflict involves those behaviors which seem to bother everyone but the exhibitor. These problems often include poor hygiene, body odors, public sexual behavior, fighting, spitting in undesignated receptacles, loud and abusive verbal behavior, property damage, begging, hoarding, constant touching, recurrent work interruptions, smoking in bed or other undesignated areas, leaving the facility without advance notice, stealing, excessive demands, continually using staff telephones, and writing or calling various "authorities" including the newspaper, relatives, governors, the President of the United States, and the FBI to report "mistreatment."

It should be recognized that most of these behaviors do not necessitate the special expertise of the clinician and will quickly occupy time which would more appropriately be used for patients' complaints. One approach would be simply for the psychologist to ignore

staff referrals but this often results in animosity or out right deprivation of patient's rights. "Time-out" rooms become holding tanks,
basic elements essential for survival become targets of response cost,
and chemicals are used to subdue target as well as nontarget responses.
In-service is the appropriate forum to acquaint personnel with more
appropriate targets for referral but the powerful effects of behavior
therapy suggest continued responsibility. When the staff has been
trained sufficiently in behavioral techniques and the performance of
these techniques is followed by positive consequences, most of these
management problems should be eliminated. By controlling the application of nonessential reinforcers such as favored foods, special
activities, television time, smoking materials, and extra social reinforcement, the nursing staff should find that management problems
become less frequent.

Extreme outbursts can often be prevented by diligent observation.
A combative episode seldom occurs with no prior, less intense
changes in behavior. Learning to recognize these changes and becoming acquainted with a patient's historical record helps to increase this
awareness. An expeditious relationship with the area mental health
center can help to minimize the impact of such episodes should they
be exhibited despite precautions.

Close observation, the rapid and consistent application of pre-
determined contingencies following problematic behavior, periodic
patient reviews, and a prompt method of referral to more appropriate
settings, should reduce concern with intense management problems.
In-service training should help to raise the threshold of acceptance
of less intense management problems through the development of
an understanding of the probable causes of such behavior. Program
design, based upon behavioral methodology, should handle the rest.

## Isolation of Potential or Actual Management Problem Cases

The presence of some or all of the management problems mentioned
above has led to a debate over the benefits of isolating potential
problem patients within a facility. Homogeneity would lead to a
variety of immediate gains for the facility staff if it were economically feasible. However, there are some serious drawbacks to complete isolation.

First, the motivation behind such isolation probably includes a desire to gain control over those patients' access to other patients and staff when problems arise. A practical objection to this desire is that nursing homes and long-term care facilities which are not licensed for psychiatric care, despite large numbers of psychiatric patients, will be in violation of the law if they utilize methods to block such access. Fire regulations, at the very least, would prevent such contingencies.

Second, despite the power of modeling effects as described elsewhere, it is highly unlikely that all predesignated problem patients would exhibit damaging behavior at the same time. Therefore, by virtue of the physical plant, some of the patients denied access to central areas of the facility would find their path blocked independent of the nature of their behavior at the time that they discovered the access blocked. Ethical implications aside, it would be highly undesirable to extinguish (or punish) appropriate or neutral behavior being exhibited by these nonproblem patients. Since it would be impractical to provide appropriate resonses to take the place of these decreased responses, inappropriate responses may result.

Third, limited access to programs which are being conducted for the rest of the facility could deprive these designated patients of valuable shaping, modeling, and restructuring situations. Conducting two (or more) activities programs would be cost-preventative.

Fourth, the stigma which would probably become attached to residing on these special wards or wings, could result in undesirable side-effects. Rehabilitation programs would be undermined by the conditioned responses of others when confronted by patients who were associated with these areas. Expectancies come to elicit self-fulfilling prophesies which may limit future rehabilitative efforts. Idiosyncratic behavior observed by others soon begins to acquire causative properties such that the overt verbalization becomes something on the order of, "Well, he acts that way *because* he's on the management ward." Ironically, given the two preceding arguments, this statement may very well become accurate.

Some elements of demarcation or isolation are desirable, however. If the facility is willing to differentially distribute their staffing patterns to allow a higher concentration on these units, potential problems may be documented and the necessary parties notified before a major episode occurs. More staff on these units along with more intense training could lead to better observation, documentation, and fewer false alarms. By keeping access to facility-wide programs free, these patients are not prevented from benefiting from necessary contacts.

It is also easier to set up smaller microcosms of behavioral programing than attempting to maintain programs throughout the entire facility. By grouping patients according to their common behavioral deficits or excesses, more continual programing is made possible. This type of operation does not violate the rights of those patients who are residing in these units while at the same time reducing the probability of infringing upon the rights of those patients who have not exhibited these difficulties in the past.

Therefore, a structural compromise is probably the most effective means of controlling potential problem patients. This compromise includes some geographic isolation for the purposes of observation and prompt intervention.

## Overcoming Inertia

Behavioral clinicians, and perhaps psychologists of all orientations will find some difficulties in attending to the needs of geriatric clients who reside in long-term care facilities. One of the first stumbling blocks which will need to be overcome is the widespread medical orientation of a majority of the potential mediators (i.e., nursing staff) and the physicians. Thorough in-service helps to alleviate those theoretical biases on the part of the nursing staff. It may be a more difficult task enlisting the requisite support of attending physicians. Both segments of the health care system are indoctrinated in the medical model and their perceptions of causality and therapeutics is heavily entrenched in organicity. While there is more and more acceptance of psychological correlates of physical disease among these groups it is generally a secondary acknowledgment which places psychological concerns subordinate to physical ones. These professionals usually identify adjustment problems, reactions to terminal illness, and grieving as being predominately psychological in nature but seldom see such concerns as more than adjunctive responses, not etiological variables. Hopefully, with the increasing sophistication of behavioral medicine technology this nearsightedness will be eroded in the future.

Once mutual respect is established between the psychological practitioner and the medical practitioner benefits for the client are increased greatly. Mutual referrals, yielding to the other's expertise, and efforts to become familiar with the other professional's language system help to increase this respect and rapport. Behaviorally oriented psychologists particularly must make an effort to educate the physician with regard to their skills and special knowledge since the preponderance of exposure which physicians receive both in training and postgraduate education is heavily laden with psychodynamic and/or psychopharmacological concepts.

The second form of inertia is also vitally important in recognizing and, if possible, overcoming. Given the economic status of many institutionalized elderly patients, many are receiving care which is reimbursed through governmental or other third-party agents. At this time, psychological evaluation and treatment, even when conducted by a licensed practicing clinical psychologist, may not be reimbursed by these third parties. This is especially the case when the psychologist is not employed by the physician. Though these agencies recognize the necessity for providing speech therapy, physical therapy, occupational therapy, and pharmacological intervention and consultation, they may not recognize nor reimburse psychotherapy. The situation is one, then, in which a population experiencing the most behavioral problems, and which can least afford to pay for treatments designed to alleviate these problems, may go untreated. Private-paying clients may be able to afford psychological intervention but there is no mechanism to pay for the same help if the client is receiving, say, Medicare-Medicaid benefits. Facilities which house nonprivate paying patients may not include such fees in their daily charges either, since these rates are subject to approval by the same agencies which have determined that psychotherapy is not a reimbursable expense on its own.

All the intrinsic or nonfinancial contingencies in the world are not likely to counter the inability of the client to pay for his or her services as conducted by a psychologist. It is ironic that the psychological orientation which can show empirically, the effectiveness of its techniques (behavior therapy), is not as likely to be provided as services provided by medically trained clinicians (psychiatrists) even though little or no valid data base is available for the latter.

State and federal psychological organizations need to make rectification of such discrepancies a high-priority goal. Nursing-home organizations and consumer groups should also concentrate their efforts on changing this system which is detrimental to the elderly. Legislative inertia and active counter-sparring by medical societies will be difficult to overcome. Stachnik's (1980) argument concerning the difficulty of changing the physician's behavior with regard to prevention of chronic illness may be equally applicable in the case of accepting psychologists as service providers.

> They [Physicians] begin their practice doing what they have been trained to do, and once begun, the contingencies of reinforcement that operated on them make it unlikely that their practice will change significantly. Without ever addressing the long-range health practices of their patients, there is a continuous supply of money, drama, prestige, and sense of accomplishment (all extremely powerful reinforcers) that maintains their current activity. (Stachnik, 1980, p. 10)

This observation is, in a general sense, not limited to the practice of medical clinicians. However, it can be clearly stated that without equal compensation, nonmedically oriented, in-patient therapy will not be voluntarily offered.

Once the contingencies for mutual referral control the behavior of both parties (probably based upon observable success), a formal or informal referral or consultation system within the facility is necessary. One successful system of referral is discussed below.

## THE REFERRAL SYSTEM

Though the encouragement of observation from all staff members is desirable, a screening mechanism is essential to limit wasted intervention time. Without an agreed upon criteria for referral, routine behavioral management problems will take up the largest percentage of referred problems.

In those cases in which no emergency exists (defined as the exhibition of behavior which is dangerous to self, others, or property), behavior which prompts a request by facility's staff should be of such a nature to suggest a dramatic change in appropriateness, a sudden onset of intensely inappropriate behavior not previously exhibited by the patient, or a gradual change in inappropriateness which has been continuing for several days or more.

Basically, nonemergency requests for psychological evaluation should be encouraged to be made only when it is deemed to be a problem which requires the special skills of a clinical psychologist. Therefore, high frequency behaviors such as residents leaving the facility against medical advice, minor disruptions, verbal abusiveness, cursing, irritability, and periodic refusals to take medicine are probably not appropriate referrals and should be handled through the knowledge and skills of other disciplines (i.e., nursing, social work, activities, administration).

All staff members are encouraged to notify the psychologist at the exhibition of self-abusive or self-injurious behavior, behavior necessitating the use of time-out, rapid deterioration in mental status or other behavior, moderate to severe depression which has been observed by the staff for several days, and changes which occur as a result of terminal illness. A physician's order should accompany such referrals unless an emergency arises in which case the order may follow intervention within 48 hours.

Problems which are referred by the attending physician for psychological assessment may be handled in a manner similar to other, nonpsychological referrals. Perforated order sheets are useful in that the original order, dated and signed by the physician, remains on the chart while a copy may be routed to the psychologist. It is good practice for the psychologist to initial and date the receipt of a physician's order on the original order or somewhere else on the patient's chart. The original order may be taken in verbal form by nursing personnel or the psychologist, such as over the telephone, to be signed by the physician as soon as possible.

The physician should be notified of the results of the intervention either in written or oral form though a written report of the results which becomes part of the chart is most desirable. This series of behaviors, from written notification to the psychologist's initialling the order to the written results being placed in the patient's chart, is helpful in meeting the requirements of outside review agencies as well as standardizing the referral system to prevent overlooked referrals. Review teams which regularly visit such facilities in an effort to monitor the quality of care for recipients of their monies place a large emphasis on record-keeping. When working with patients who are receiving third-party reimbursement, even though there is no mechanism for direct reimbursement, it is quite easy to become overwhelmed with the requirements for notation and documentation. A balance between such documentation and adequate delivery of care is oftentimes difficult to establish. Ironically, the facility psychologist is placed in a position in which his or her services are neither recognized nor reimbursed, yet he or she will have these services reviewed and regulated.

Many of the arguments for the necessity of a psychologist, particularly with a behavioral orientation, in nursing homes are the same as those presented in the next chapter concerning geriatric psychology in general. It is surprising that, given the ready availability, the controlled environment, and the need, more behavioral researchers have not addressed the issues which are relevant to long-term care. Like the field of aging in general, special problems and possibilities exist which are peculiar to this type of client. It is far less surprising, however, given the financial condition of these facilities, the lack of reimbursement, and the existence of the medical bias, that very few behavioral *clinicians* are involved.

# 10

# An Argument for a Behavioral Perspective in Clinical Geriatrics

Behavioral intervention with its theoretical origins in experimental psychology and its continued use backed by experimental verification is no longer content to fight for acceptance by arguing against traditional therapies. In the early years, a rather loyal and vociferous group of pioneers spent a lot of time citing data which empirically dealt significant blows to such cherished traditions as projective tests, nondirective therapists, symptom substitution in nondynamic therapy (Yates, 1958), and even the efficacy of treatment (Eysenck, 1952).

Objections to historically accepted approaches does not automatically invoke an unbounded embrace of the new approach, however. Once comparisons between approaches prove the relative superiority of one method over another, the very act of comparison becomes absurd. Not only does such activity appear to be overly defensive (to borrow an expression) but the logic is questionable. Once one method is proven to be of limited effectiveness, little can be gained by the comparison of new methods to that criterion. So we, as behavior therapists and/or researchers, moved on into another arena which involved the verification of internal processes within the methodology. The prevalence of professional journals, organizations, papers, poster sessions and behaviorally oriented training programs attest to the fact that this second-stage analysis has also proven successful.

While continued efforts to polish methodology will always be followed by positive consequences, entry into the next stage of verification is imperative. Methodological refinements are important but it is now time to become more problem-oriented. The age-related dysfunctions previously addressed offer such a test of behavioral methodology in a new problem area.

This population, even through the traditional therapist's eyes, presents problems which are most effectively treated directly, with little attention to restructuring entire "personalities." In this instance, the bias regarding differential treatment of the elderly has left a positive effect. Instead of attempting to alter the dynamics thought to underlie maladaptive behavioral signs, most clinicians realize, at least with the elderly, that such reorganization through insight is unnecessary. A point that behavior therapists have contended since the beginning. With attention on behavior rather than intrapsychic dynamics most clinicians dealing with geriatric patients have become, in effect, behaviorists. Support for a complete behavioral perspective is provided by the components or corollaries of behavior theory.

## SHORT-TERM THERAPY

The emphasis on short-term nonintrapsychic treatment encourages the utilization of behavior therapy. Schaie and Schaie (1977, p. 715) address this issue.

> In contrast to a similar analysis with younger clients, it is important to recognize that what is required is not a description of basic personality patterns as such, since no profound personality reorganization is likely to be attempted. Thus, much more emphasis will likely be given to state than trait variables.

It is important to note that the motivation behind the use of short-term therapy and the emphasis on state factors is not due to the fact that clinicians expect a short duration between intervention and death. This consideration should not enter into the clinical picture at all. However, therapists should identify with specific target behaviors (Pfeiffer & Busse, 1973) and resources (Brink, 1978), because this appoach has a high probability of meeting with success. The emphasis on selecting *behavior* as the target for change fits directly into the expertise of those who have followed this perspective from the start.

## MINIMIZING INFERENCES

A direct corollary of the theoretical approach described above is the desire to limit the number of inferences made from observable behavior to primary cause. Behavior theory has always declined to rely on inferential stages. Employing more inferences leads to a reliance on unseen, immeasurable constructs and, as a result, a lengthier therapeutic process. A hypothetical illustration may help to clarify this difference.

Consider a situation in which you are seated in a patient dining room in a long-term care facility. You notice an elderly woman propelling herself in a geriatric chair in the general direction of a large window overlooking the grounds. She is moving in a jerky fashion as her chair catches up with each new placement of her feet. A variety of inferences may be made regarding this peculiar behavior depending upon the orientation of the observer. The variability in the inferences involves the distance one's willing to go (or has to go) from the description of the observed behavior to the hypothesis regarding its cause. For instance, a developmental stage-theorist might make the observation that such behavior resembles a preambulatory child's locomotor behavior and, thus, he or she is witness to age-induced regression. A psychodynamic practitioner would probably see symbolic masturbation or the search for a lost-symbolized love object. A clinical pharmacist would spot a special type of drug side-effect (akathisia) due to long-term phenothiazine use. Meanwhile the behaviorist would confidently observe a patient directing herself toward a source of (sensory) reinforcement.

These views differ in their acceptability basically because they vary greatly in their propensity for empirical validation. Let us suppose that we were to continue our observation of this elderly lady a while longer. Instead of continuing in the path toward the window, she veers off, and proceeds to go around a dining table a dozen or so times. Is the behaviorist's hypothesis in the most trouble since it is the only one which considered external control over the observed behavior? Is the fact that the behaviorist must now shift the "motivation" to, say, a form of self-stimulatory behavior, mean that his or her approach is the least valuable? The behaviorist would contend that just the opposite were true. The argument is that the behaviorst typically tenders the most testable (and rejectable) hypotheses from which to work and therefore wastes less time in inappropriate intervention and nomothetic explanations of behavior. The first two observers are locked into their inferences while the third, though far more testable, depends upon some of the same observational and empirical techniques as behavior therapy (e.g., reversal designs, time-sampling methodology, using the subject as his or her own control), but typically does not utilize them.

The dependency on inferences is a tricky circumstance. We are seldom aware just how much of our thinking about a client's behavior involves inferences. We would probably fare better if we described the behavior observed, described the events preceding and following the behavior, and left it at that.

## FUNCTIONAL ANALYSIS

The act of viewing behavior as a function of preceding and consequential events, a major theoretical corollary of behavior theory, is also a valuable methodological approach to the problems of aging. It is also closely tied with the ideas described above. If we are to take the elderly's behavior at face value (though not necessarily independent of less readily available indices) the possible etiological factors become more predictable. For example, given the knowledge of severely disrupted sensation, memory impairment, and a nonstimulating environment (antecedent variables) and consequence variables such as deficits in reinforcement for alternative behavior, it is not difficult to predict the nature of the response. The "equation" works equally well given an unknown quantity at any point in the model if sufficient information is provided regarding the other two quantities. From such an analysis we may then proceed from prediction of response to a fairly accurate formulation for control of response. If we can control or manipulate aspects of the model at either the antecedent or consequent points, we should expect to observe predicted changes in the nature of the response itself. If we permit ourselves to work within a model which emphasizes the relationship between observable behavior and, say, the lunar phases or some underlying personality trait, we set ourselves up for a very difficult time in terms of predicting changes in behavior observed across situations or within a given cycle of lunar phase.

Behavior is simply a function of its antecedents and consequences, the consequences quickly becoming antecedents for further behavior. We may find that the behavior observed in geriatric patients is a function of antecedents and consequences not frequently addressed by behaviorists (e.g., hypoglycemia, cerebrovascular accidents, relocation) but the analysis is the same.

## DE-EMPHASIZING CATEGORIZATION

Behavior therapists are disinclined to communicate with category labels offered by the majority of practitioners and reinforced by lay persons and sources of reimbursement. A description or summary of observed behavior which takes the form of a list of problematic responses, although more time-consuming, makes the task of treatment validation much easier. It should also be noted that such "problem-oriented" descriptions are being promoted more now by regulatory agencies to be used in planning of patient care. It has now become evident that such agencies deliver aversive consequences to facilities which continue the practice of equating problem areas with diagnoses. This rather powerful contingency favors descriptions which behaviorally oriented clinicians also favor. It is not simply a matter of a change in verbal behavior, however, since it has long been recognized that standard diagnostic labels not only have low reliability and validity but may also be iatrogenic. Practitioners who use more descriptive accounts of problematic responding should find it less difficult to accommodate this enlightened approach.

For example, professionals who are used to describing behavior in language such as, "Disorientation to time and place due to severe memory dysfunction secondary to long-term alcohol abuse and recent relocation" rather than as, "Chronic organic brain syndrome with Wernicke's features," should have less difficulty in fitting into the new model espoused by these agencies. It is also the case that care-providers can carry out special treatment plans much easier. The less ambiguously stated is the actual problem, the more consistent the delivery of care.

## THE EXPERIMENTAL-CLINICAL APPROACH

The fact that clinical technique as applied to the problems of the aged is a relatively new development, substantial support for specific methodologies is lacking. The typical procedure, if we were to be guided by traditional verification paradigms, would be to study the relative effectiveness of established techniques on a readily assessable sample of elderly persons in fairly controlled settings. Certain subsamples would be chosen randomly to receive X treatment, another Y, and so on, while one group would serve as a control. However, there are only a few academic complexes which contain both individuals skilled in outcome research and a significant sample of elderly patients. There are few ready-made "guinea pigs" such as those enrolled in introductory psychology classes who are often involved in research projects conducted by faculty or graduate students. As a matter of fact, the limitations of analogue research may demand more direct access to clinically relevant problems anyway. The truly significant problems which make up most of clinical intervention and which need most immediate attention are present in samples of elderly persons not inclined to participate in or to have access to research projects. Rather than settling for less than representative samples of subjects, problems, and techniques, an approach which simultaneously attends to clinical application and experimental concerns is favored, particularly for those behaviors which are extremely bizarre, intense or troublesome (i.e., interesting) and less likely to be found in traditional research-oriented settings.

Behavior therapists are trained to attend to treatment variables during direct application. The use of reversal designs, using the client as his or her own control, and alternating treatments within one subject are a few of the approaches which are increasingly being recognized as powerful treatment-evaluation tools. Though group designs which employ highly desirable controls for internal validity are very valuable, single subject designs, with sufficient replications across subjects and sufficient reversals within a subject may be more practical. Given the susceptibility to attentional factors alone, baseline and a return-to-baseline phases alternated systematically with the treatment of choice, would help to reveal treatment effects over and above attentional benefits. Since many of the elderly who exhibit behavior problems are receiving medication, the drug level may also be used as the baseline against which behavior therapy effects may be evaluated.

The combination of experimental and clinical behavior is a relatively new approach and one which is common only to psychologists trained in applied-clinical methodology. Treating every client as a miniexperiment[1] is typically emphasized only during the training of behavior therapists.

A final point should be made with regard to this idea of combining empirical testing with application. It is unlikely that compensatory behavior can accurately be displayed and assessed in situations which differ greatly from those situations which the elderly are likely to encounter. In other words, contrived situations which are designed by the experimenter/therapist to evoke compensatory behavior are probably not realistic enough to yield valid results. However, taking the research to the places in which such a response is likely to occur (e.g., nursing homes, mental health clinics) increases the validity of one's statements regarding treatment efficacy.

## SYSTEM DESIGN AND BEHAVIORAL ENGINEERING

In their excellent article, Baltes and Barton (1977) suggest, among other things, the need to approach the problems of the elderly from the operant or biobehavioral model. They advocate the utilization of reinforcement and stimulus modification procedures in order to develop environments which are conducive for adequate response. Behavioral technology, unlike the applied techniques of most other psychological approaches, can be used in total systems design. The successful application of operant techniques discussed in Chapter 7

---

[1] This approach should not be construed as advocating experimentation with naive clients solely for the benefit of the therapist's professional aspirations. "Experimental" as used here suggests the need for continual monitoring of those variables which effect the outcome of treatment.

may be effectively applied to an entire population of elderly individuals housed in a common residence. Behavioral technology also offers systematized observation and documentation procedures which are easily taught to persons in constant contact with the clients. The relationship is a mutualistic one. Those clinicians who apply behavior technology depend upon the environment to maintain these technologies and those who interact daily with elderly clients may have to depend upon sound behavioral technology in order to make their jobs easier.

Behavioral techniques may be incorporated into the designs of new living environments or in the modification of existing structures. For several recent descriptions of behaviorally designed settings, the reader is referred to Beattie (1970), DeLong (1974), Lawton (1977), McClannahan (1973), and Risley and Edwards (1978), among others.

## TRAINING OF MEDIATORS AND OBSERVERS

The settings in which most of the problematic behavior occurs make it not only convenient, but necessary, to include existing staff as mediators, data collectors, observers, and evaluators. These skills are encouraged within a behavioral approach in two ways. First, the staff are more involved in many behavioral programs than with other "private" psychotherapies. Since the modification of behavior of an elderly client, as with any other client, is seen by the behavioral clinician as being directly affected by environmental antecedents and consequences, the staff or families who are part of, or control, these variables are ideal modifiers of target responses. Second, behavioral technology provides a language which is more easily understandable than the language of psychodynamics. Training in data recording, the breakdown of molar behaviors into smaller measurable responses, and the analysis of interactions between the client and various aspects of his or her environment, are all presented in simple and directly applicable behavioral-terminology.

The "common sense" theoretical principles and the simplicity of application of most of the behavioral programs encourages the use of mediators particularly, but not exclusively, with institutionalized geriatric patients. Attention to these points is certainly within the realm of nursing responsibilities throughout all levels of the nursing hierarchy. The breakdown of responses into small increments also promotes treatment effectiveness and, as a result, reinforces the mediator's participation in the treatment program. The effectiveness of the programs per se in relatively short time-spans also serves to encourage future cooperation on the part of these mediators.

Some of the components of behavioral programming may also be useful in other areas of the management of elderly clients. Charting and documentation procedures require brief, concise, and operationally sound observations in order to promote communication among health care providers. The SOAP and DAP problem strategies for recording the providers' assessment, observations, and treatment plans, though not established by behavior therapists, certainly incorporate principles which agree with behavioral procedures and language.

In patient care-planning, the probability that program ideas will follow smoothly from the statement of the problem and that measurable goals will be described, increases if the problems are stated, unambiguously, and in increments. These incremental steps are easily monitored and yield valuable information regarding progress. Behavioral technicians who are used to stating problems in these terms are quite familiar with the benefits of accurately stated care-plans. For instance, instead of stating that a given patient is "Claustrophobic" the problem may be stated as, "Experiences severe (or moderate, or mild) anxiety within 100 feet (or 10, or 1) of an elevator." This leads to a more easily evaluated target once an intervention is chosen. In other words, the complete documentation of the parameters of the response, a description of the intervention, and the method of evaluation of that intervention is most desirable. This is the language of the behavior therapist.

## ETHICS AND ACCOUNTABILITY

It should not be argued that age necessarily dictates the special need for protection of third parties, but it can be accurately stated that, for multiple reasons, many elderly individuals needing treatment are unable to perceive noneffective or detrimental procedures. Whether the problem involves a lack of sophistication in psychotherapeutic techniques, a lack of general assertiveness, or general incompetency brought about by some of the changes described in earlier chapters, accountability of treatment application may not be accurately assessed by the client. For this reason, one should favor the use of intervention techniques which not only work but which also include the keeping of data which easily support this effectiveness on an individual basis. This does not, of course, mean that each elderly client who receives psychotherapy must make his/her problem or treatment known to the public. However, should a question arise either from the client or an interested and responsible third party, the data and description of progress and procedures is readily presentable. Publication of the results of these procedures helps to further the field of gerontology and promotes replication.

The behavioral approach generally encourages such accountability. Again, we are not arguing that clinicians who do not practice from a behavioral mode are incompetent or devious. It is simply that anyone else who does business in any other field of endeavor is encouraged to document procedures in the handling of, say, their business affairs. It is not a matter of personal ethics or professionalism, it is a question of the consequences that continued practice with noneffective techniques has on a person's life.

## CONTINUITY ACROSS THE LIFE-SPAN

The concepts used within a behavioral framework such as response parameters, functional analysis, stimulus control and response competency, are theoretically the same regardless of the age of the client or the nature of the behavior exhibited (Smyer & Gatz, 1979). As these principles hold for the development and maintenance of normal as well as abnormal behavior, they hold true for any organism's behavior regardless of age. Those involved in the new field of behavioral pediatrics have in no way found it necessary to ascribe to qualitatively different concepts. They have, like those in behavioral geriatrics, found it necessary only to offer typological modifications which fit within the concepts previously formulated.

The application of a functional analysis of behavior, the principles of reinforcement, and the modification of behavior through the manipulation of controlling contingencies are still important even though the functional analysis may need expansion, the reinforcers need reconsideration, and the contingencies may be different. What we are suggesting is not the development of new theory but rather the development of age-specific considerations in the application of existing theory. By minimizing discontinuity in the approach regardless of the age of the individual, it is hoped that attention will be focused on more relevant issues.

## BEHAVIOR THEORY AND THE COMPENSATORY MODEL

Finally, the acceptance of a new descriptive model of aging based upon behavior as a response to naturally occurring age-related phenomena, exists well within a behavioral approach. Not only may behavior theory and its applications be used to define compensatory behavior and the strategies necessary for the appropriate development of constructive compensation, but they both share a very fundamental optimism regarding the clinical picture in geriatric psychology. Viewing most of the behavioral manifestations of inappropriate geriatric behavior as inappropriate compensatory response suggests *modifiability*. Such a description of a preponderance of abnormal responding found with this population is incompatible with a therapeutic approach which assumes crystallization or rigidity in elderly response. Behavior theory makes no comment on the inflexibility of responding in this age group, it simply provides valid strategies for changing behavior. Where certain manifestations exist which are not subject to external manipulations, both the model and the theory may still be applied to the excess pathological responses, i.e., the responses to the organically induced responses.

Put simply, there are no elderly individuals, no matter how debilitated, who do not exhibit some responses which may be modified and these modifications should help to alleviate at least a part of the discomfort. There should be no preconceived notions as to how far one can go even with "unreachable" individuals. There are no cases where *nothing* can be done. We owe it to ourselves, our clients, and the population as a whole to keep this idea foremost in our activities.

# Appendix A
## Mental Status Evaluation

Patient _____    Room _____

Age and D.O.B. _____    Assessor _____

Date and Time _____

I. Please write completely the patient's responses to the following:

   1. What is the name of this place? _____

   2. What is today's date (day of month)? _____

   3. What month is it? _____

   4. What is the year? _____

   5. How old are you? _____

   6. When is your birthday? _____

   7. When were you born? _____

   8. Who is the President of the United States? _____

   9. Who was the President before him? _____

II. Now tell the patient to remember these three items: *chair, door, tree.* Ask the patient to repeat these items. Response: _____
Ask again about three minutes later.

III. Record in the appropriate spaces below those descriptors which most accurately describe this patient's behavior. Add any descriptors which may not be listed where appropriate.

**217**

1. APPEARANCE AND BEHAVIOR
   a. Posture _____
   b. Gait (loping, shuffling, etc.) _____
   c. Grooming (hair brushed, tidy clothes, cleaniness, etc.) _____
      _____
   d. Tics or tremors _____
   e. Motor behavior _____
      (Lethargy, restlessness, calm and composed, lack of spontaneous movement, rigidity, stereotyped movements, picking at body, grimacing, etc.)
   f. Additional observations: _____
      _____

2. SPEECH_____
   (Rapid, slow, pressured, monotonous, loud, mute, whispered, stuttering, spontaneous, unintelligible, perseveration, loose associations, etc.)

3. THOUGHT _____
   _____
   (Delusions, obsessions, frequent complaints, hallucinations, suicidal, blocking, flight of ideas, rambling, normal, etc.)

4. MOOD AND AFFECT (The emotional state of the patient and how they
   say they feel)_____
   _____
   (Sad, hostile, suspicious, angry, apathetic, guilty, normal, flat, irritable, tense, depressed, defensive, unreal, etc.)

5. At about this point, ask for the aforementioned memory items. Response:
   _____

6. Ask the patient to repeat the following numbers in the same order that you give them. Instruct the patient not to respond until all of the numbers in one series are given.
   a. 5–8–2 _____   b. 6–9–4 _____   c. 6–4–3–9 _____
   d. 7–2–8–6 _____   e. 4–2–7–3–1_____
   f. 7–5–8–3–6 _____ ___

Now instruct the patient to give the numbers backward.

a. 2–4 _____     b. 5–8 _____     c. 6–2–9 _____

d. 4–1–5 _____     e. 3–2–7–9 _____ f. 4–9–6–8 _____

(Please note: Stop after two failures of the same length)

7. Briefly, give your impressions of the way the patient related to you during this evaluation (Friendly, hostile, uncooperative, cooperative, etc.)

_____

_____

_____

8. DISPOSITION (To be completed by the psychologist): _____

_____

_____

_____

_____

_____

_____

9. Follow-up #1 _____

_____

Follow-up #2 _____

_____

Follow-up #3 _____

_____

# Appendix B
## Examination for Behavior Therapy In-Service

1. Behavior therapy has its roots in which of the following disciplines:

   (a) Psychoanalysis
   (b) Medicine
   (c) Experimental Psychology
   (d) Psychosurgery

2. A low-frequency appropriate behavior is the target for a behavioral program. Which basic principle is true regarding plans to increase the frequency of that behavior:

   (a) Ignore the behavior when it occurs
   (b) Place the patient in the "time-out" room following the occurrence of such behavior
   (c) Follow the occurrence of the behavior with an aversive event
   (d) Follow the occurrence of the behavior with something positive

3. Which of the following procedural statements is NOT true regarding the use of a "time-out" room:

   (a) Twenty minutes is the absolute maximum time that a patient can spend in the room at any one time
   (b) A physician's order must accompany the use of the room
   (c) Only those patients who are predesignated may be placed in the room
   (d) The patient should be checked midway through the time-out period

4. Where may the program plans, such as the urinary incontinence program, be found:

   (a) On the chart cover
   (b) On the patient's door
   (c) In the central nursing Kardex at the nursing station
   (d) On the bulletin board behind the nursing station

5. Which of the following tend to be high frequency stopping places for "wanderers" in this facility:

   (a) Cannot be determined the behavior is random
   (b) Isolated areas
   (c) Windows with exterior views
   (d) Sources of reinforcement such as water fountains and food trays

6. What is the best way to handle the "extinction phenomenon" described in class:

   (a) Consider using punishment in conjunction with the extinction program
   (b) Terminate the program and seek an order for medication
   (c) Lengthen the period of "time-out" to one hour for each occurrence of inappropriate behavior
   (d) Have patience and continue observing and recording the behavior

7. When you observe sudden confusion, disorientation, and extreme agitation in an elderly patient with no prior history of such behavior which causative variable would you suspect first:

   (a) Infantile impulses
   (b) An acute physical or drug problem.
   (c) Senile dementia
   (d) Sudden release of previously denied masturbatory fantasies

8. Observations of decreased appetite, late onset sleep, and a general slowing are suggestive of which of the following problems:

   (a) Organic mental disorder     (c) Depression
   (b) Sexual dysfunction          (d) Paranoia

9. Behavior therapy tends to place less emphasis on which of the following variables:

   (a) Early childhood
   (b) Irrational thinking on the part of the client
   (c) Conditioning principles
   (d) The effects of environmental consequences on behavior

10. Which one of the following physical problems is least likely to be accompanied by behavioral problems:

    (a) Diabetes mellitus          (c) Cerebrovascular accidents
    (b) Arthritis                  (d) Cerebroarteriosclerosis

The case description which follows is to be referred to while answering questions 11 through 15.

A 72-year-old female patient has recently been admitted to this facility from an acute care hospital. She has a history of one psychiatric admission twenty-two years previously which resulted in a two-month stay and a diagnosis of schizophrenia, simple type. She has advanced cataracts bilaterally, diabetes mellitus, periodic reactions to insulin and poor hearing and is currently receiving Diazepam, NPH Insulin, and Hydergine®. The Diazepam given for 4½ years is decreased to one-half the dose on admission. After she has been in the facility two days, she suddenly becomes extremely confused, agitated, and restless. She reports having vivid nightmares and addresses persons not existing in reality.

11. Which of the following is probably not a cause of the current manifestations in this patient:

    (a) Withdrawal of the Diazepam
    (b) Schizophrenia
    (c) Sensory impairment and isolation
    (d) Insulin reaction

12. During the observation period which of the following would not be targets for recording:

    (a) Symbolic content of the nightmares
    (b) Amount of food consumed
    (c) Routine blood sugar levels
    (d) Time of day and number of hallucinations

13. Which of the following is LEAST likely to cause the problems described above:

    (a) Recent relocation                  (c) Insulin
    (b) Hydergine®                         (d) Sensory deprivation

14. One built-in method in our facility for assessing the change in this person's mental status is:

    (a) CT scan                            (c) Depression inventory
    (b) Rorshach inkblot test              (d) Mental Status Evaluation

15. Which therapeutic approach would NOT be indicated in the future when the patient has been stabilized:

    (a) Routine blood sugar levels
    (b) Education in the nature and treatment of diabetes
    (c) Phenothiazine regimen
    (d) Relaxation training to reduce anxiety

16. In behavioral interventions it is often desirable to record the behavior of interest prior to intervention. This phase is called:

    (a) Reversal phase                     (c) Treatment phase
    (b) Baseline phase                     (d) Control phase

17. The schedule of reinforcement delivery in which not every desired response is followed by reinforcement is called:

    (a) Extinction
    (b) Intermittent reinforcement

(c) Primary reinforcement

(d) Continuous reinforcement

18. If a patient cannot verbally indicate potential rewards to be used in behavior therapy, how could you go about finding out what could be used:

  (a) Present all possible reinforcements to the patient until he or she responds

  (b) Unfortunately, there is nothing that can be done

  (c) Use a punishment design instead

  (d) Observe the patient and use items or activities which the patient spontaneously engages in.

19. Which of the following procedures DO NOT fall under the realm of behavior therapy:

  (a) Electroshock therapy (EST)      (c) Modeling

  (b) Shaping                         (d) "Time-out"

20. Which of the following would be useful counter-responses to train to replace anxiety-responding:

  (a) Laughter or crying

  (b) Relaxation or coping statements

  (c) Coping statements or avoidance

  (d) Avoidance or sleep

21. Perhaps the most reliable differentiating index between organic and functional disorders is:

  (a) Intensity of the behavior

  (b) Onset of the behavior

  (c) Duration of the behavior

  (d) Number of medications currently being taken

22. The behaviorist would prefer not using such diagnostic labels as organic mental disorder and schizophrenia but rather prefers:

  (a) Ignoring the symptom complexes involved

  (b) Using the term organic brain syndrome

  (c) Looking at the observable behaviors which usually go into making up such a diagnosis

  (d) Analyzing the underlying causes of such behavior

23. The therapy which involves modification of attitudes and inappropriate thinking is called:

  (a) Psychoanalysis

  (b) Gestalt therapy

  (c) Systematic desensitization

  (d) Rational restructuring

24. Which of the following statements is NOT true with regard to the principles of reinforcement aimed at increasing a response:

(a) The reinforcer should be delivered immediately following the response
(b) The reinforcer should be given continuously after each response so designated
(c) Everyone who has contact with the patient should be aware of the targeted response
(d) The reinforcer should be only in the form of water or food.

25. The most frequent psychological problem among the elderly is:

(a) Alzheimer's disease
(b) Depression
(c) Schizophrenia, chronic undifferentiated type
(d) Involutional melancholia

Note: The answers to the Behavior In-Service Examination are as follows: 1. c, 2. d, 3. d, 4. a, 5. c, 6. d, 7. c, 8. c, 9. a, 10. b, 11. b, 12. a, 13. b, 14. d, 15. c, 16. b, 17. b, 18. d, 19. a, 20. b, 21. b, 22. c, 23. d, 24. d, 25. a.

# Bibliography

Abrahams, J. P., Wallach, H. F., and Divens, S. 1979. Behavioral improvement in long-term geriatric patients during an age-integrated psychosocial rehabilitation program. *Journal of the American Geriatric Society,* **27**, 218–221.

Adams, R. A., and Victor, M. 1970. Delirium and other confusional states and Korsakoff's amnestic syndrome. *In,* M. M. Wintrobe *et al.* (eds.), *Harrison's Principles of Internal Medicine, 6th Edition.* New York: McGraw-Hill Book Company.

Agras, W. S., Kazdin, A. E., and Wilson, G. T. 1979. *Behavior Therapy: Toward An Applied Clinical Science.* San Francisco: W. H. Freeman and Company.

Altman, H., Mehta, D., Evenson, R. C., and Sletten, I. W. 1973. Behavioral effects of drug therapy on psychogeriatric inpatients. I. Chlorpromazine and thioridazine. *Journal of the American Geriatric Society,* **21**, 241–248.

Anders, T. R., and Fozard, J. L. 1973. Effects of age upon retrieval from primary and secondary memory. *Developmental Psychology,* **9**, 411–415.

Anderson, B., and Palmore, E. 1974. Longitudinal evaluation of ocular function. *In,* E. Palmore (ed.), *Normal Aging.* Durham, North Carolina: Duke University Press.

Angel, R. W. 1977. Understanding and diagnosing senile dementia. *Geriatrics,* **32**, 47–49.

Appleton, W. S. 1976. Third psychoactive drug usage guide. *Diseases of the Nervous System,* **37**, 39–51.

Arenberg, D. 1968. Concept problem solving in young and old adults. *Journal of Gerontology,* **23**, 279–282.

Arenberg, D. 1965. Anticipation interval and age differences in verbal learning. *Journal of Abnormal Psychology,* **70**, 419–425.

Arenberg, D. 1973. Cognition and aging: verbal learning, memory, problem solving, and aging. *In,* C. Eisdorfer and M. P. Lawton (eds.), *The Psychology of Adult Development and Aging.* Washington, D.C.: American Psychological Association.

Atthowe, J. M. 1972. Controlling nocturnal enuresis in severely disabled and chronic patients. *Behavior Therapy,* 3, 232–239.

Back, K. W., and Gergen, K. J. 1966. Cognitive and motivational factors in aging and disengagement. *In,* I. H. Simpson and J. C. McKinney (eds.), *Social Aspects of Aging.* Durham, North Carolina: Duke University Press.

Bahrick, H. P., Bahrick, P. O., and Wittlinger, R. P. 1975. Fifty years of memory for names and faces: a cross-sectional approach. *Journal of Experimental Psychology: General,* 104, 54–75.

Baltes, M. M., and Barton, E. M. 1977. New approaches toward aging: a case for the operant model. *Educational Gerontology: An International Quarterly,* 2, 383–405.

Barash, D. P. 1977. *Sociobiology and Behavior.* New York: Elsevier.

Barnes, J. A. 1974. Effects of reality orientation classroom on memory loss confusion and disorientation in geriatric patients. *Gerontologist,* 14, 138–142.

Barns, E. K., Sack, A., and Shore, H. 1973. Guidelines to treatment approaches. *Gerontologist,* 13, 513–527.

Bassuk, E. L., and Schoonover, S. C. 1977. *The Practitioner's Guide to Psycho-active Drugs.* New York: Plenum Medical Book Company.

Beattie, W. M. 1970. The design of supportive environments for the life-span. *Gerontologist,* 10, 190–193.

Beck, A. T., Ward, C. H., Mendelson, M., Mock, J., and Erbaugh, J. 1961. An inventory for measuring depression. *Archives of General Psychiatry,* 4, 561–571.

Benson, D. F. 1974. Normal pressure hydrocephalus: a controversial entity. *Geriatrics,* 29, 125–132.

Berger, R. M., and Rose, S. D. 1977. Interpersonal skill training with institutionalized elderly patients. *Journal of Gerontology,* 32, 346–353.

Berkowitz, S. 1978. Informed consent, research, and the elderly. *Gerontologist,* 18, 237–243.

Berry, R. G. 1975. Pathology of dementia. *In,* J. G. Howells (ed.), *Modern Perspectives in the Psychiatry of Old Age.* New York: Brunner/Mazel, Publishers.

Bijou, S. W., Peterson, R. F., Harris, F. R., Allen, K. E., and Johnston, M. S. 1969. Methodology for experimental studies of young children in natural settings. *The Psychological Record,* 19, 177–210.

Birkhill, W. R., and Schaie, K. W. 1975. The effect of differential reinforcement of cautiousness in intellectual performance among the elderly. *Journal of Gerontology,* 30, 578–583.

Birren, J. E. 1970. Toward an experimental psychology of aging. *American Psychologist,* 25, 124–135.

Birren, J. E., Butler, R. N., Greenhouse, S. W., Sokoloff, L., and Yarrow, M. R. 1963. *Human aging.* (UAPHA No. 986). Washington, D.C.: United States Public Health Service.

Blackman, D. K. 1977. Control of urinary incontinence among the institutionalized elderly. Paper presented at the 11th Annual Convention of the Association for the Advancement of Behavior Therapy, Atlanta, Georgia.

Bondareff, W. 1977. The neural basis of aging. *In*, J. E. Birren and K. W. Schaie (eds.), *Handbook of the Psychology of Aging.* New York: Van Nostrand Reinhold Company.

Bondareff, W., Narotzky, R., and Routtenberg, A. 1971. Intrastriatal spread of catecholamines in senescent rats. *Journal of Gerontology,* **26**, 163–167.

Botwinick, J. 1966. Cautiousness in advanced age. *Journal of Gerontology,* **21**, 347–353.

Botwinick, J. 1967. *Cognitive Processes in Maturity and Old Age.* New York: Springer Publishing Company, Inc.

Botwinick, J. 1973. *Aging and Behavior.* New York: Springer Publishing Company, Inc.

Botwinick, J. 1969. Disinclination to venture responses versus cautiousness in responding: age differences. *Journal of Genetic Psychology,* **115**, 55–62.

Botwinick, J., and Kornetsky, C. 1960. Age differences in the acquisition and extinction of the GSR. *Journal of Gerontology,* **15**, 83–84.

Brezinski, W., Jones, E. A., Atkinson, D., and Noah, J. C. 1977. Senior citizens integration project: a self-care, self-sufficiency behavioral systems program for institutionalized geriatric residents. Paper presented at the Association for the Advancement of Behavior Therapy, Atlanta, Georgia.

Brink, T. L. 1978. Geriatric rigidity and its psychotherapeutic implications. *Journal of the American Geriatric Society,* **26**, 274–277.

Brink, T. L., Belanger, J., Bryant, J., Capri, D., Janakes, C., Jasculca, S., and Oliveira, C. 1978. Hypochondriasis in an institutional geriatric population: construction of a scale (HSIG). *Journal of the American Geriatric Society,* **26**, 557–559.

Brink, T. L., Capri, D., DeNeeve, V., Janakes, C., and Oliveira, C. 1979. Hypochondriasis and paranoia: Similar delusional systems in an institutionalized geriatric population. *Journal of Nervous and Mental Disease,* **167**, 224–236.

Brody, E. M., Kleban, M. H., Lawton, M. P., and Silverman, H. A. 1971. Excess disabilities of mentally impaired aged: Impact of individualized treatment. *Gerontologist,* **11**, 124–133.

Brook, P., Degan, G., and Mather, M. 1975. Reality orientation, a therapy for psychogeriatric patients: a controlled study. *British Journal of Psychiatry,* **127**, 42–45.

Bruning, R. H., Holzbauer, I., and Kimberlin, C. 1975. Age, word imagery, and delay interval: Effects on short-term and long-term retention. *Journal of Gerontology,* **30**, 312–318.

Bry, P. M., and Nawas, M. M. 1969. Rigidity: A function of reinforcement history. *Perceptual and Motor Skills,* **29**, 118.

Buchanan, D. S. 1978. Iatrogenic causes of neurologic disorders: Part 2. Drug-related dysfunctions. *Geriatrics,* **33**, (9), 47–52.

Burnet, M. 1974. *Intrinsic Mutagenesis: A Genetic Approach to Ageing.* New York: John Wiley & Sons.

Busse, E. W. 1976. Hypochondriasis in the elderly: a reaction to social stress. *Journal of the American Geriatric Society,* **24**, 145–149.

Busse, E. W., and Pfeiffer, E. (eds). 1969. *Behavior and Adaptation in Late Life.* Boston: Little, Brown.

Canestrari, R. E. 1963. Paced and self-paced learning in young and elderly adults. *Journal of Gerontology,* 18, 165–168.

Cautela, J. R. 1972. Manipulation of the psychosocial environment of the geriatric patient. *In,* D. P. Kent, *et al.* (eds.), *Research Planning and Action for the Elderly: The Power and Potential of Social Science.* New York: Behavioral Publications.

Cautela, J. R., and Kastenbaum, R. A. 1967. Reinforcement Survey Schedule for use in therapy, training, and research. *Psychological Reports,* 20, 1115–1130.

Chapron, D., and Lawson, I. 1978. Drug prescribing and care of the elderly. *In,* W. Reichel (ed.), *Clinical Aspects of Aging.* Baltimore: The Williams & Wilkins Company.

Citrin, R. S., and Dixon, D. N. 1977. Reality orientation: a milieu therapy used in an institution for the aged. *Gerontologist,* 17, 39–43.

Coleman, K. K. 1963. The modification of rigidity in geriatric patients through operant conditioning. *Dissertation Abstracts,* 24, 2560–2561.

Copeland, J. R. M., Kelleher, M. J. Kellet, J. M., Gourlay, A. J., Gurland, B. J., Fleiss, J. L., and Sharpe, L. 1976. A semi-structured clinical interview for the assessment of diagnosis and mental state in the elderly: The Geriatric Mental Status Schedule. *Psychological Medicine,* 6, 439–449.

Corke, P. O. 1964. Complex behavior in "old" and "young" rats. *Psychological Reports,* 15, 371–376.

Cornbleth, T. 1977. Effects of a protected hospital ward area on wandering and nonwandering geriatric patients. *Journal of Gerontology,* 32, 573–577.

Corso, J. F. 1977. Auditory perception and communication. *In,* J. E. Birren and K. W. Schaie (eds.), *Handbook of the Psychology of Aging.* New York: Van Nostrand Reinhold Company.

Craik, F. I. M. 1977. Age differences in human memory. *In,* J. E. Birren and K. W. Schaie (eds.), *Handbook of the Psychology of Aging.* New York: Van Nostrand Reinhold Company.

Crook, T. H. 1979. Psychometric assessment in the elderly. *In,* A. Raskin and L. F. Jarvik (eds.), *Psychiatric Symptoms and Cognitive Loss in the Elderly.* New York: John Wiley & Sons.

Crovitz, B. 1966. Recovering a learning deficit in the aged. *Journal of Gerontology,* 21, 236–238.

Davies, D. R., and Griew, S. 1965. Age and vigilance. *In,* A. T. Welford and J. E. Birren (eds.), *Behavior, Aging, and the Nervous System.* Springfield, Ill.: Charles C. Thomas.

DeLong, A. J. 1974. Environments for the elderly. *Journal of Communication,* 24, 101–112.

Diamond, M. C. 1978. The aging brain: some enlightening and optimistic results. *American Scientist,* 65, 66–71.

Dibner, A. S. 1975. The psychology of normal aging. *In*, M. G. Spencer and C. J. Dorr (eds.), *Understanding Aging: A Multidisciplinary Approach*. New York: Appleton-Century-Crofts.

Di Mascio, A., and Sovner, R. D. 1976. Neuroleptic-induced extrapyramidal side effects: a plan for rational treatment. *Drug Therapy*, 6, 99–103.

Doty, B. A., and Doty, L. A. 1964. Effect of age and chlorpromazine on memory consolidation. *Journal of Comparative and Physiological Psychology*, 57, 331–334.

Drummond, L., Kirchhoff, L., and Scarbrough, D. R. 1978. A practical guide to reality-orientation: A treatment approach for confusion and disorientation. *Gerontologist*, 18, 568–573.

D'Zurilla, T. J., and Goldfried, M. R. 1971. Problem-solving and behavior modification. *Journal of Abnormal Psychology*, 78, 107–126.

Eisdorfer, C., and Cohen, D. 1978. The cognitively impaired elderly: differential diagnosis. *In*, M. Storandt, I. C. Sigler, and M. F. Elias (eds.), *The Clinical Psychology of Aging*. New York: Plenum Press.

Epstein, L. J. 1976. Symposium on age differentiation in depressive illness. *Journal of Gerontology*, 31, 278–282.

Epstein, L. J. 1978. Clinical geropsychiatry. *In*, W. Reichel (ed.), *Clinical Aspects of Aging*. Baltimore: The Williams and Wilkins Company.

Ernst, P., Badash, D., Beran, B., Kosovsky, R., and Kleinhauz, M. 1977. Incidence of mental illness in the aged: unmasking the effects of a diagnosis of chronic brain syndrome. *Journal of the American Geriatric Society*, 25, 371–375.

Ernst, P., Beran, B., Badash, D., Kosovsky, R., and Kleinhauz, M. 1977. Treatment of the aged mentally ill: further unmasking of the effects of a diagnosis of chronic brain syndrome. *Journal of the American Geriatric Society*, 25, 466–469.

Ernst, P., Beran, B., and Kleinhauz, M. 1979. Dr. Ernst and his colleagues reply. *Gerontologist*, 19, 530–533.

Ernst, P., Beran, B., Safford, F., and Kleinhauz, M. 1978. Isolation and the symptoms of chronic brain syndrome. *Gerontologist*, 18, 468–474.

Eysenck, H. J. 1952. The effects of psychotherapy: An evaluation. *Journal of Consulting Psychology*, 16, 319–325.

Fassler, L. B., and Gaviria, M. 1978. Depression in old age. *Journal of the American Geriatric Society*, 26, 471–475.

Fishback, D. B. 1977. Mental status questionnaire for organic brain syndrome with a new visual counting test. *Journal of the American Geriatric Society*, 25, 167–170.

Fleiss, J., Gurland, B., and Des Roche, P. 1976. Distinctions between organic brain syndrome and functional psychiatric disorders. *International Journal of Aging and Human Development*, 7, 323–330.

Folsom, J. C. 1968. Reality orientation for the elderly mental patient. *Journal of Geriatric Psychiatry*, 1, 291–307.

Fox, J. H., Topel, J. L., and Huckman, M. S. 1975. Dementia in the elderly: a search for treatable illnesses. *Journal of Gerontology*, **30**, 557–564.

Fozard, J. L., Wolf, E., Bell, B., McFarland, R. A., and Podolsky, S. 1977. Visual perception and communication. *In*, J. E. Birren and K. W. Schaie (eds.), *Handbook of the Psychology of Aging*. New York: Van Nostrand Reinhold Company.

Frolkis, V. V. 1977. Aging of the autonomic nervous system. *In* J. E. Birren and K. W. Schaie (eds.), *Handbook of the Psychology of Aging*. New York: Van Nostrand Reinhold Company.

Garrison, J. E. 1978. Stress management training for the elderly: a psychoeducational approach. *Journal of the American Geriatric Society*, **26**, 397–403.

Geiger, O. G., and Johnson, L. A. 1974. Positive education for elderly persons. *Gerontologist*, **14**, 432–436.

Glass, C. R., Gottman, J. M., and Shmurak, S. H. 1976. Response acquisition and cognitive self-statement modification approaches to dating skills. *Journal of Counseling Psychology*, **23**, 520–526.

Glassman, A. H., Bigger, J. T., Jr., Giardina, E. V., Kantor, S. J., Perel, J. M., and Davies, M. 1979. Clinical characteristics of imipramine-induced orthostatic hypotension. *Lancet*, **1**. 8114, 468–472.

Goldfried, M. R., and Davison, G. C. 1976. *Clinical Behavior Therapy*. New York: Holt, Rinehart & Winston.

Goldfried, M. R., and D'Zurilla, T. J. 1969. A behavioral-analytic model for assessing competence. *In*, C. D. Spielberger (ed.), *Current Topics in Clinical and Community Psychology, Volume 1*. New York: Academic Press.

Goldfried, M. R., and Goldfried, A. P. 1975. Cognitive change methods. *In*, F. H. Kanfer and A. P. Goldstein (eds.), *Helping People Change*. New York: Pergamon Press.

Goldstein, S. E. 1979. Depression in the elderly. *Journal of the American Geriatric Society*, **27**, 38–42.

Goodrick, C. L. 1968. Learning, retention, and extinction of a complex maze habit for mature-young and senescent Wistar albino rats. *Journal of Gerontology*, **23**, 298–304.

Goulet, L. R. 1972. New directions for research on aging and retention. *Journal of Gerontology*, **27**, 52–60.

Gurland, B. J. 1976. The comparative frequency of depression in various adult age groups. *Journal of Gerontology*, **31**, 283–292.

Gurland, B. J., Copeland, J., Sharpe, L., and Kelleher, M. 1976. The Geriatric Mental Status interview (GMS). *International Journal of Aging and Human Development*, **7**, 303–311.

Hachinski, V. C., Lassen, N. A., and Marshall, J. 1974. Multi-infarct dementia: a cause of mental deterioration in the elderly. *Lancet*, **2**, 207–210.

Haglund, R. M. J., and Schuckit, M. A. 1976. A clinical comparison of tests of organicity in elderly patients. *Journal of Gerontology*, **31**, 654–659.

Hall, R. C. W., Cruzenski, W. P., and Popkin, M. K. 1979. Differential diagnosis of somatopsychic disorders. *Psychosomatics*, **20**, 381–389.

Hamilton, W. D. 1964. The genetical theory of social behaviour: I. and II. *Journal of Theoretical Biology*, 7, 1–52.

Hansten, P. D. 1976. *Drug Interactions*. Philadelphia: Lea & Febiger.

Havighurst, R. J. 1968. A social-psychological perspective on aging. *Gerontologist*, 8, 67–71.

Hayflick, L. 1968. Human cells and aging. *Scientific American*, 218, 32–37.

Hayflick, L. 1977. The biology of aging. *Natural History*, 86, 22–33.

Hersch, E. L. 1979. Development and application of the extended scale for dementia. *Journal of the American Geriatric Society*, 27, 348–354.

Hersen, M., and Barlow, D. H. 1976. *Single-Case Experimental Designs: Strategies for Studying Behavior Change*. New York: Pergamon Press.

Hertzog, C. K., Williams, M. V., and Walsh, D. A. 1976. The effect of practice on age differences in central perceptual processing. *Journal of Gerontology*, 31, 428–433.

Hogstel, M. O. 1979. Use of reality orientation with aging confused patients. *Nursing Research*, 28, 161–165.

Hontela, S., and Schwartz, G. 1979. Myocardial infarction in the differential diagnosis of dementias in the elderly. *Journal of the American Geriatric Society*, 27, 104–106.

Howell, S. C. 1972. Familiarity and complexity in perceptual recognition. *Journal of Gerontology*, 27, 364–371.

Hoyer, W. J. 1973. Application of operant techniques to the modification of elderly behavior. *Gerontologist*, 13, 18–22.

Hoyer, W. J., Kafer, R. A., Simpson, S. C., and Hoyer, F. W. 1974. Reinstatement of verbal behavior in elderly mental patients using operant procedures. *Gerontologist*, 14, 149–152.

Hughes, C. P., Myers, F. K., Smith, K., and Libow, L. S. 1973. Pseudosenility: acute and reversible organic brain syndromes. *Journal of the American Geriatric Society*, 21, 112–120.

Hulicka, I. M., and Grossman, J. L. 1967. Age-group comparisons for the use of mediators in paired-associate learning. *Journal of Gerontology*, 22, 46–51.

Hulicka, I. M., and Weiss, R. L. 1965. Age differences in retention as a function of learning. *Journal of Consulting Psychology*, 29, 125–129.

Hussian, R. A. 1979. The combination of operant and cognitive therapy with geriatric patients. Paper presented at the Association for Behavior Analysis, Dearborn, Michigan.

Hussian, R. A., and Hill, S. D. 1980. Stereotyped behavior in elderly patients with chronic organic mental disorder. *Journal of Gerontology*, 35, 689–691.

Hussian, R. A., and Lawrence, P. S. 1981, in press. Social reinforcement of activity and problem-solving training in the treatment of depressed institutionalized elderly patients. *Cognitive Therapy and Research*, 1981, in press.

Hussian, R. A. 1980, submitted to *Behavior Therapy*. Stimulus control in the modification of problematic behavior in elderly institutionalized patients.

Hyerstoy, B. J. 1979. The role of a psychologist in a nursing home. *Professional Psychology*, 10, 36–41.

Jani, S. N. 1966. The age factor in stereopsis screening. *American Journal of Optometry*, **43**, 653–655.

Jarvik, L. F., and Cohen, D. 1973. A biobehavioral approach to intellectual change with aging. *In*, C. Eisdorfer and M. P. Lawton (eds.), *The Psychology of Adult Development and Aging*. Washington, D.C.: American Psychological Association.

Jenkins, J., Felce, D., Lunt, B., and Powell, L. 1977. Increasing engagement in activity of residents in old people's homes by providing recreational material. *Behavior Research and Therapy*, **15**, 429–434.

Jeste, D. V., Potkin, S. G., Sinha, S., Feder, S., and Wyatt, R. J. 1979. Tardive dyskinesia—reversible and persistent. *Archives of General Psychiatry*, **36**, 585–590.

Johnson, D. M., Parrott, G. L., and Stratton, R. P. 1968. Production and judgment of solutions to five problems. *Journal of Educational Psychology*, **59**, Part 2, 1–21.

Jones, E. A., Brown, K., Noah, J. C., Atkinson-Jones, D., and Brezinski, W. 1977. Three behavioral strategies to increase participation in leisure time activities in institutionalized geriatric populations. Paper presented at the Association for the Advancement of Behavior Therapy, Atlanta, Georgia.

Karoly, P. 1975. Operant methods. *In*, F. H. Kanfer and A. P. Goldstein (eds.), *Helping People Change: A Textbook of Methods*. New York: Pergamon Press.

Kastenbaum, R., and Sherwood, S. 1972. VIRO: A scale for assessing the interview behavior of elderly people. *In*, D. P. Kent, R. Kastenbaum, and S. Sherwood (eds.), *Research Planning and Actions for the Elderly*. New York: Behavioral Publications.

Kelleher, M., Copeland, J., Gurland, B., and Sharpe, L. 1976. Assessment of the older psychiatric inpatient. *International Journal of Aging and Human Development*, **7**, 295–302.

Kenshalo, D. R. 1977. Age changes in touch, vibration, temperature, kinesthesis and pain sensitivity. *In*, J. E. Birren and K. W. Schaie, *Handbook of the Psychology of Aging*. New York: Van Nostrand Reinhold Company.

Kent, D. P., Kastenbaum, R., and Sherwood, S. (eds.). 1972. *Research Planning and Actions for the Elderly*. New York: Behavioral Publications.

Kent, S. 1977. Classifying and treating organic brain syndromes. *Geriatrics*, **32**, 87–96.

Killian, J. 1970. Effects of geriatric transfers on mortality rates. *Social Work*, **15**, 19–26.

Kochansky, G. E. 1979. Psychiatric rating scales for assessing psychopathology in the elderly: a critical review. *In*, A. Raskin and L. F. Jarvik (eds.), *Psychiatric Symptoms and Cognitive Loss in the Elderly*. New York: John Wiley & Sons.

Korsgaard, S., and Skavsig, O. B. 1979. Increase in weight after treatment with depot neuroleptics. *Acta Psychiatrica Scandinavica*, **59**, 139–144.

Kousler, D. H., and Kleim, D. M. 1978. Age differences in processing relevant versus irrelevant stimuli in multiple-item recognition learning. *Journal of Gerontology*, 33, 87–93.

Kubany, E. S., and Sloggett, B. B. 1973. Coding procedure for teachers. *Journal of Applied Behavior Analysis*, 6, 339–344.

Labouvie-Vief, G., and Gonda, J. N. 1976. Cognitive strategy training and intellectual performance in the elderly. *Journal of Gerontology*, 31, 327–332.

Langer, E., Janis, I., and Wolfer, J. 1975. Reduction of psychological stress in surgical patients. *Journal of Experimental Social Psychology*, 11, 155–165.

Langer, E. J., Rodin, J., Beck, P., Weinman, C., and Spitzer, L. 1978. Environmental determinants of memory improvement in late adulthood. Unpublished manuscript, Harvard University.

Laurence, M. W. 1967. Memory loss with age: a test of two strategies for its retardation. *Psychonomic Science*, 9, 209–210.

Lawson, J. S., Rodenburg, M., and Dykes, J. A. 1977. A dementia rating scale for use with psychogeriatric patients. *Journal of Gerontology*, 32, 153–159.

Lawton, M. P. 1972. Assessing the competence of older people. *In*, D. P. Kent, R. Kastenbaum, and S. Sherwood (eds.), *Research Planning and Actions for the Elderly*. New York: Behavioral Publications.

Lawton, M. P. 1972. The dimensions of morale. *In*, D. P. Kent, R. Kastenbaum, and S. Sherwood (eds.), *Research Planning and Actions for the Elderly*. New York: Behavioral Publications.

Lawton, M. P. 1977. The impact of the environment on aging and behavior. *In*, J. E. Birren and K. W. Schaie (eds.), *Handbook of the Psychology of Aging*. New York: Van Nostrand Reinhold Company.

Lawton, M. P., and Brody, E. M. 1969. Assessment of older people: self-maintaining and instrumental activities of daily living. *Gerontologist*, 9, 179–186.

Lawton, M. P., and Nahemow, L. 1973. Ecology and the aging process. *In*, C. Eisdorfer and M. P. Lawton (eds.), *The Psychology of Adult Development and Aging*. Washington, D.C.: American Psychological Association.

Lawton, P., and Yaffe, S. 1970. Mortality, morbidity, and voluntary change of residence by older people. *Journal of the American Geriatric Society*, 18, 823–831.

Leaf, A. 1973. Getting old. *Scientific American*, 229, 45–52.

Lee, D. 1969. An adjunct to training psychiatric aides in behavior modification techniques. *Journal of Psychiatric Nursing and Mental Health Services*, 7, 169–171.

Letcher, P. B., Peterson, L. P., and Scarbrough, D. 1974. Reality orientation: a historical study of patient progress. *Hospital and Community Psychiatry*, 25, 801–803.

Lewisohn, P. M., and Graf, M. 1973. Pleasant activities and depression. *Journal of Consulting and Clinical Psychology*, 41, 261–268.

Libb, J. W., and Clements, C. B. 1969. Token reinforcement in an exercise program for hospitalized geriatric patients. *Perceptual and Motor Skills*, 28, 957–958.

Libow, L. S. 1973. Pseudo-senility: acute and reversible organic brain syndromes. *Journal of the American Geriatric Society*, 21, 112-120.

Libow, L. S. 1977. Senile dementia and "pseudosenility": clinical diagnosis. *In*, C. Eisdorfer and R. O. Friedel (eds.), *Cognitive and Emotional Disturbances in the Elderly*. Chicago: Year Book Medical Publishers, Inc.

Lieberman, M. A. 1975. Adaptive processes in late life. In, N. Datan and L. H. Ginsberg (eds.), *Life-span Developmental Psychology*. New York: Academic Press.

Linn, M. W. 1967. A rapid disability rating scale. *Journal of the American Geriatric Society*, 15, 211-214.

Linski, N., Howe, M. W., and Pinkston, E. M. 1975. Behavioral group work in a home for the aged. *Social Work*, 20, 454-463.

Lipton, M. A. 1976. Age differentiation in depression: Biochemical aspects. *Journal of Gerontology*, 31, 293-299.

MacDonald, M. L. 1973. The forgotten Americans: a sociopsychological analysis of aging and nursing homes. *American Journal of Community Psychology*, 1, 272-294.

MacDonald, M. L. 1976. The ethics of using behavior modification with the institutionalized aging: a practical analysis. *Journal of Long-Term Care Administration*, 4, 42-46.

MacDonald, M. L. 1978. Environmental programming for the socially isolated aging. *Gerontologist*, 18, 350-354.

MacDonald, M. L., and Butler, A. K. 1974. Reversal of helplessness: Producing walking behavior in nursing home wheelchair residents using behavior modification procedures. *Journal of Gerontology*, 29, 97-101.

MacDonald, M. L., and Settin, J. M. 1978. Reality orientation versus sheltered workshops as treatment for the institutionalized aging. *Journal of Gerontology*, 33, 416-421.

Masoro, E. 1972. Other physiologic changes with age. *In*, A. M. Ostfeld and D. C. Gebsch (eds.), *Epidemiology of Aging*. (NIH) 77-711. Elkridge, Maryland: U.S. Dept. of HEW.

McAllister, C. J., Scowden, E. B., and Stone, W. J. 1978. Toxic psychosis induced by phenothiazine administration in patients with chronic renal failure. *Clinical Nephrology*, 10, 191-195.

McClannahan, L. E. 1973. Therapeutic and prosthetic living environments for nursing home residents. *Gerontologist*, 13, 424-429.

McClannahan, L. E., and Risley, T. R. 1975. Design of living environments for nursing-home residents: increasing participation in recreation activities. *Journal of Applied Behavior Analysis*, 8, 261-268.

Meer, B., and Baker, J. A. 1966. The Stockton Geriatric rating scale. *Journal of Gerontology*, 21, 392-403.

Meichenbaum, D. 1972. Cognitive modification of test anxious college students. *Journal of Consulting and Clinical Psychology*, 39, 370-380.

Meichenbaum, D. 1973. Therapist manual for cognitive behavior modification. Unpublished manuscript, University of Waterloo.

Meichenbaum, D. 1977. *Cognitive-Behavior Modification.* New York: Plenum Press.

Meichenbaum, D., and Turk, D. C. 1976. The cognitive-behavioral management of anxiety, anger, and pain. *In,* P. Davidson (ed.), *The Behavioral Management of Anxiety, Depression and Pain.* New York: Brunner/Mazel.

Mendlewicz, J. 1976. The age factor in depressive illness: some genetic considerations. *Journal of Gerontology,* **31**, 300–303.

Mishara, B. L. 1978. Geriatric patients who improve in token economy and general milieu treatment programs: a multivariate analysis. *Journal of Consulting Clinical Psychology,* **46**, 1340–1348.

Monge, R., and Hultsch, D. 1971. Paired-associate learning as a function of adult age and length of the anticipation and inspection intervals. *Journal of Gerontology,* **26**, 157–162.

Moos, R. H. 1974. Psychological techniques in the assessment of adaptive behavior. *In,* G. V. Coelho, D. A. Hamburg, and J. E. Adams (eds.), *Coping and Adaptation.* New York: Basic Books, Inc., Publishers.

Mueller, D. J., and Atlas, L. 1972. Resocialization of regressed elderly residents: a behavioral management approach. *Journal of Gerontology,* **27**, 390–392.

National Institute of Health. Special report on aging: 1979. (NIH Pub. No. 79–1907) Washington, D.C.: United States Government Printing Office, 1979.

Novaco, R. W. 1975. *Anger Control: The Development and Evaluation of an Experimental Treatment.* Lexington, Massachusetts: D. C. Heath, Lexington Books.

Nursing home care in the United States: Failure in public policy. 1974. Introductory report, subcommittee on long-term care of the special committee on aging, United States Senate, 93rd Congress. Washington, D.C.: U.S. Government Printing Office.

Oberleder, M. 1966. Psychotherapy with the aging: an art of the possible? *Psychotherapy: Theory, Research and Practice,* **3**, 139–142.

Obrist, W. D., Busse, E. W., Eisdorfer, C., and Kleemeier, R. W. 1962. Relation of the electroencephalogram to intellectual function in senescence. *Journal of Gerontology,* **17**, 197–206.

O'Neil, P. M., and Calhoun, K. S. 1975. Sensory deficits and behavioral deterioration in senescence. *Journal of Abnormal Psychology,* **84**, 579–582.

Oster, C. 1979. Sensory deprivation and homeostasis. *Journal of the American Geriatric Society,* **24**, 461–464.

Oster, C. 1979. Sensory deprivation and homeostasis. *Journal of the American Geriatric Society,* **27**, 364–367.

Parker, B., Deibler, S., Feldshuh, B., Frosch, W., Laureana, E., and Sitten, J. 1976. Finding medical reasons for psychiatric behavior. *Geriatrics,* 1976, **31** (6), 87–91.

Parnes, S. J. 1967. *Creative Behavior Guidebook.* New York: Charles Scribner's Sons.

Peak, D. 1972. Psychiatric problems of the elderly seen in an outpatient clinic.

*In,* E. Pfeiffer (ed.), *Alternatives to institutional care for older Americans: Practice and Planning.* National Conference on Alternatives to Institutional Care for Older Americans, Duke University.

Pfeiffer, E. 1972. Designing systems of care: The clinical perspective. *In,* E. Pfeiffer (ed.), *Alternatives to institutional care for older Americans: Practice and Planning.* National Conference on Alternatives to Institutional Care for Older Americans, Duke University.

Pfeiffer, E. 1975. A short portable mental status questionnaire for the assessment of organic brain deficit in elderly patients. *Journal of the American Geriatric Society,* **23,** 433–441.

Pfeiffer, E., and Busse, E. W. 1969. Mental disorders in later life—affective disorders; paranoid, neurotic, and situational reactions. *In,* E. Busse and E. Pfeiffer (eds.), *Behavior and Adaptation in Late Life.* Boston: Little, Brown.

Pfeiffer, E., and Busse, E. W. 1973. Mental disorders in later life—affective disorders, paranoid, neurotic, and situational reactions. *In,* E. W. Busse and E. Pfeiffer (eds.), *Mental Illness in Later Life.* Washington, D.C.: APA.

Pino, C. J., Rosica, L. M., and Carter, T. J. 1978. The differential effects of relocation on nursing home patients. *Gerontologist,* **18,** 167–172.

Powell, R. R. 1974. Psychological effects of exercise therapy upon institutionalized geriatric mental patients. *Journal of Gerontology,* **29,** 157–161.

Quilitch, H. R. 1974. Purposeful activity increased on a geriatric ward through programmed recreation. *Journal of the American Geriatric Society,* **22,** 226–229.

Rabbitt, P. 1968. Age and the use of structure in transmitted information. *In,* G. A. Talland (ed.), *Human Aging and Behavior.* New York: Academic Press.

Reichel, W. 1978. The evaluation of the confused, disoriented, or demented elderly patient. *In,* W. Reichel (ed.), *Clinical Aspects of Aging.* Baltimore, Maryland: The Williams & Wilkins Company.

Rinke, C. L., Williams, J. J., Lloyd, K. E., and Smith-Scott, W. 1978. The effects of prompting and reinforcement on self-bathing by elderly residents of a nursing home. *Behavior Therapy,* **9,** 873–881.

Risley, T. R., and Edwards, K. A. 1978. Behavioral techniques for nursing home care: toward a system of nursing home organization and management. First annual Nova Behavioral Conference on Aging, Port St. Lucie, Florida.

Rockstein, M. 1958. Heredity and longevity in the animal kingdom. *Journal of Gerontology,* Supplement No. 2, **13,** 7–12.

Rodin, J., and Langer, E. J. 1977. Long-term effects of a control-relevant intervention with the institutionalized aged. *Journal of Personality and Social Psychology,* **35,** 897–902.

Rodstein, M., and Oei, L. S. 1979. Cardiovascular side effects of long-term therapy with tricyclic antidepressants in the aged. *Journal of the American Geriatric Society,* **27,** 231–234.

Rossman, I. 1978. Clinical assessment in geriatrics. From proceedings of a National Conference: *Assessment and Evaluation Strategies in Aging: People,*

*Populations, and Programs.* G. L. Maddox, Chair, Duke University Center for the Study of Aging and Human Development.

Rover, C. K., Cohen, R. Y., and Shlapack, W. 1975. Life span stability in olfactory sensitivity. *Developmental Psychology,* 11, 311–318.

Salzman, C., and Shader, R. I. 1978. Depression in the elderly: I. Relationship between depression, psychologic defense mechanisms, and physical illness. *Journal of the American Geriatric Society,* 26, 253–258.

Salzman, C., and Shader, R. I. 1979. Clinical evaluation of depression in the elderly. *In,* A. Raskin and L. F. Jarvik (eds.), *Psychiatric Symptoms and Cognitive Loss in the Elderly.* New York: John Wiley & Sons.

Salzman, C., Shader, R. I., Kochansky, G. E., and Cronin, D. M. 1972. Rating scales for psychotropic drug research with geriatric patients. I. Behavior ratings. *Journal of the American Geriatric Society,* 20, 209–214.

Schaie, K. W., and Schaie, J. P. 1977. Clinical assessment and aging. *In,* J. E. Birren and K. W. Schaie (eds.), *Handbook of the Psychology of Aging.* New York: Van Nostrand Reinhold Company.

Schaie, K. W., and Strother, C. R. 1968. Cognitive variables in older college graduates. *In,* G. A. Talland (ed.), *Human Aging and Behavior.* New York: Academic Press.

Schwartz, A. N., and Peterson, J. A. 1979. *Introduction to Gerontology.* New York: Holt, Rinehart and Winston.

Schwenk, M. A. 1979. Reality orientation for the institutionalized aged: does it help? *Gerontologist,* 19, 373–377.

Sekhon, S. S., and Maxwell, D. S. 1974. Ultra-structural changes in neurons of the spinal anterior horn of aging mice with particular reference to the accumulation of lipofuscin pigment. *Journal of Neurocytology,* 3, 59–72.

Shmavonian, B. M., Miller, L. H., and Cohen, S. I. 1968. Differences among age and sex groups in electro-dermal conditioning. *Psychophysiology,* 5, 119–131.

Sinex, F. M. 1975. The biochemistry of aging. *In,* M. G. Spencer and C. J. Dorr (eds.), *Understanding Aging: A Multidisciplinary Approach.* New York: Appleton-Century-Crofts, 1975.

Sinnott, J. D. 1977. Sex-role inconstancy, biology, and successful aging: a dialectical model. *Gerontologist,* 17, 459–463.

Smith, A. D. 1975. Aging and interference with memory. *Journal of Gerontology,* 30, 319–325.

Smith, B. J., and Barker, H. R., Jr. 1972. Influence of a reality orientation training program on the attitudes of trainees toward the elderly. *Gerontologist,* 12, 262–264.

Smyer, M. A., and Gatz, M. 1979. Aging and mental health: Business as usual. *American Psychologist,* 34, 240–246.

Smyer, M. A., Hofland, B. F., and Jonas, E. A. 1979. Validity study of the short portable mental status questionnaire for the elderly. *Journal of the American Geriatric Society,* 27, 263–269.

Spangler, P. F., Edwards, K. A., and Risley, T. R. 1977. Behavioral care of non-ambulatory geriatric patients. Association for the Advancement of Behavior Therapy, Atlanta, Georgia.

Sparacino, J. 1978. An attributional approach to psychotherapy with the aged. *Journal of the American Geriatric Society*, 26, 414–417.

Spencer, M. G., and Dorr, C. J. (eds.). 1975. *Understanding Aging: A Multidisciplinary Approach*. New York: Appleton-Century-Crofts.

Stachnik, T. J. 1980. Priorities for psychology in medical education and health care delivery. *American Psychologist*, 35, 8–15.

Steel, K. 1978. Evaluation of the geriatric patient. *In*, W. Reichel (ed.), *Clinical Aspects of Aging*. Baltimore, Maryland: The Williams & Wilkins Company.

Strehler, B. L. 1961. Studies on the comparative physiology of aging. II: On the mechanism of temperature life-shortening in *drosophilia melanogaster*. *Journal of Gerontology*, 16, 2–12.

Strehler, B. L. 1977. *Time, Cells, and Aging*. New York: Academic Press.

Stroot, V. R., Lee, C. A., and Schaper, C. A. 1975. *Fluids and Electrolytes: A Practical Approach*. Philadelphia: F. A. Davis Company.

Surwillo, W. W. 1968. Timing of behavior in senescence and the role of the CNS. *In*, G. A. Talland (ed.), *Human Aging and Behavior*. New York: Academic Press.

Taub, H. A. 1975. Mode of presentation, age, and short-term memory. *Journal of Gerontology*, 30, 56–59.

Thompson, L. W. 1976. Cerebral blood flow, EEG, and behavior in aging. *In*, R. D. Terry and S. Gershon (eds.), *Aging. Vol. 3: Neurobiology of Aging*. New York: Raven Press.

Thompson, L. W., and Marsh, G. R. 1973. Psychophysiological studies of aging. *In*, C. Eisdorfer and M. P. Lawton (eds.), *The Psychology of Adult Development and Aging*. Washington, D.C.: American Psychological Association.

Timiras, P. S. 1972. *Developmental Physiology and Aging*. New York: The Macmillan Company.

Toseland, R., and Rose, S. D. 1978. A social skills training program for older adults: evaluation of three group approaches. *Social Work Research Abstracts*.

Turk, D. C. 1978. Application of coping-skills training to the treatment of pain. *In*, C. D. Spielberger and I. G. Sarason (eds.), *Stress and Anxiety* (Vol. 5). New York: Brunner/Mazel.

Ullman, L. P., and Krasner, L. 1969. *A Psychological Approach to Abnormal Behavior*. Englewood Cliffs, New Jersey: Prentice-Hall, Inc.

Van Der Kolk, B. A. 1978. Organic problems in the aged: brain syndromes and alcoholism, introduction. *Journal of Geriatric Psychiatry*, 11, 131–134.

Van Scheyen, J. D., and Van Kammen, D. P. 1979. Clomipramine-induced mania in unipolar depression. *Archives of General Psychiatry*, 36, 560–565.

Verwoerdt, A. 1976. *Clinical Geropsychiatry*. Baltimore, Maryland: The Williams & Wilkins Company.

Vickers, R. 1976. The therapeutic milieu and the older depressed patient. *Journal of Gerontology*, 31, 314–317.

Walsh, A. C. 1976. Hypochondriasis associated with organic brain syndrome: A new approach to therapy. *Journal of the American Geriatric Society*, **24**, 430–431.

Walsh, D. A., and Thompson, L. W. 1978. Age differences in visual sensory memory. *Journal of Gerontology*, **33**, 383–387.

Wang, H. S. 1973. Special diagnostic procedures—the evaluation of brain impairment. *In*, E. W. Busse and E. Pfeiffer (eds.), *Mental Illness in Later Life*. Washington, D.C.: American Psychiatric Association.

Wang, H. S., and Busse, E. W. 1969. EEG of healthy old persons—a longitudinal study: I. Dominant background activity and occipital rhythm. *Journal of Gerontology*, **24**, 419–426.

Warren, L. R., Wagener, J. W., and Herman, G. E. 1978. Binaural analysis in the aging audition system. *Journal of Gerontology*, **33**, 731–736.

Waugh, N. C., Thomas, J. C., and Fozard, J. L. 1978. Retrieval time from different memory stores. *Journal of Gerontology*, **33**, 718–724.

Welford, A. T., and Birren, J. E. (eds). 1965. *Behavior, Aging, and the Nervous System*. Springfield, Illinois: Charles C. Thomas.

Wells, C. E. 1976. Delirium and dementia. *In*, H. Abrams (ed.), *Basic Psychiatry for the Primary Care Physician*. Boston: Little, Brown.

Whitlock, F., and Evan, L. 1978. Drugs and depression. *Drugs*, **15**, 53–71.

Willner, M. 1978. Individual psychotherapy with the depressed elderly outpatient: An overview. *Journal of the American Geriatric Society*, **26**, 231–235.

Wine, I. 1970. Investigations of attentional interpretation of test anxiety. Unpublished doctoral dissertation, University of Waterloo.

Wisniewski, H. M., and Terry, R. D. 1976. Neuropathology of the aging brain. *In*, R. D. Terry and S. Gershon (eds.), *Aging. Vol. 3: Neurobiology of Aging*. New York: Raven Press.

Wisocki, P. A., and Mosher, P. 1980. Peer-facilitated sign language training for a geriatric stroke victim with chronic brain damage. *Journal of Geriatric Psychiatry*, **13**, 89–102.

Witte, K. L., and Freund, J. S. 1976. Paired-associate learning in young and old adults as related to stimulus concreteness and presentation method. *Journal of Gerontology*, **31**, 186–192.

Wittkower, E. D., and Warnes, H. 1977. *Psychosomatic Medicine*. Hagerstown, Maryland: Harper & Row, Publishers.

Wolpe, J. 1969. *The Practice of Behavior Therapy*. New York: Pergamon Press.

Wotring, K. E. 1978. Problems in management: Diabetes in the psychiatric patient. *Journal of Psychiatric Nursing*, **16** (8), 26–28.

Yates, A. J. 1958. The application of learning theory to the treatment of tics. *Journal of Abnormal and Social Psychology*, **56**, 175–182.

Yesavage, J. 1979. Dementia: Differential diagnosis and treatment. *Geriatrics*, **34**, 51–62.

Zarit, S. H. 1979. Helping an aging patient to cope with memory problems. *Geriatrics*, **34**, 82–90.

# Index

Life Satisfaction Scale, 132
Lipofuscin, 13, 14

Mediators, 189–190, 212–213
Medication: assessment, 113, 188–189; non-psychoactive drugs, 54, 59, 61–63; psychotropics, 53–59, 178–179; toxicity, 59, 62; as treatment, 176–177
Meditation, 170
Memory, 5–9: dichotic, 6; elimination of defects, 7–8, 9, 161; impairment of, 69, 72, 78, 88; incidental, 6; paired-associate tasks, 6; pictorial, 8; primary, 6–7; rote learning and, 6; secondary, 7
Memory-for-Designs, 137
Mental Status Exam, 217–219: and acute organic changes, 66–69; and chronic organic change, 75–76, 78–79
Milieu therapy, 180
Modeling: and self-instructional training, 34; therapy, 177–178, 181–182, 185
Modified reality orientation, 132–134

Neologisms: and chronic organic changes, 74, 81
Nurses Observation Scale for Inpatient Evaluation (NOSIE), 137

Oberleder Attitude Scale, 131
Operant conditioning, 5: acquisition, 5; extinction, 5; magnification in, 48; perseveration, 5; rigidity and, 5, 8–9; therapy, 133, 164–168
Organic Brain Syndrome. See Acute organic changes and Chronic organic changes
Organic Mental Disorder. See Acute organic changes and Chronic organic changes

Paranoid behavior: assessment, 97–98; modeling, 178; and organic processes, 51, 54, 60, 64; response to changes, 23, 95; symptoms, 95–97; and transition, 39; treatment, 175–176
Parkinsonism: and anxiety, 102; and drugs, 54, 55
Perception. See Sensation and perception
Personality: changes in, 64, 69, 72; as target, 206
Physical Self-Maintenance Scale (PSMS), 105
Physical therapy, 101, 136, 201
Physiological changes, 12–16: autonomic nervous system, 13–14; central nervous system, 14–15; connective tissues, 13; lipofuscin, 13, 14; and pharmacokinetics, 53; and sensory deprivation, 135–136

Problem-solving training, 35–39: and compensatory model, 38–39; in coping, 162–163; procedure, 36–38; in social skills training, 159–160; and transition, 38
Psychosomatic illness, 52

Rapid Disability Rating Scale, 78–79
Rational restructuring: with paranoid behavior, 175–176
Raven's Progressive Matrices Test, 137–138, 162
Reality orientation: and acute organic disorders, 125; and chronic organic dysfunction, 129–132; modified, 132–135; versus sheltered workshop, 131–132; and staff behavior, 131; training, 189
Reality Orientation Information Sheet (ROIS), 130
Reciprocal altruism. See Altruistic behavior
Referral, 201, 202–204
Reimbursement, 186, 201–202, 204, 209–210
Reinforcement: and activity level, 136–137; and ambulation, 154–155; and depression, 164–168; and exercise, 137–138; and incontinence, 142; measuring, 117; principles, 188; and self-feeding, 153; and self-stimulation, 147; and sexual behavior, 145–146; and skills loss, 153; sources of, 48, 198; and verbal behavior, 155–158; and wandering, 140–141
Reinforcement Survey Schedule, 117
Relaxation training, 54: for anxiety, 170; for paranoid behavior, 175; in stress-inoculation training, 42; in systematic desensitization, 40
Relocation: and depression, 90; and problem-solving training, 38; and sensory deprivation, 86, 87, 169; treatment, 181–182, and unassertiveness, 177
Resocialization, 155, 158, 161
Rigidity: on complex tasks, 12; in intellectual performance, 8–9; and limited stimuli, 21; and memory, 8; and operant conditioning, 5, 12

Secondary gain, 100
Self-care, 180
Self-feeding skills, 153–154
Self-instructional training, 41–43, 162–163
Self-statements: in depression, 94, 167–168; negative, 34–35, 42, 126; in paranoid behavior, 95–96, 175–176; in self-instructional training, 34, 162–163; in stress-inoculation training, 42–43, 172–